NATIONAL ACADEMIES *Sciences Engineering Medicine*

NATIONAL ACADEMIES PRESS
Washington, DC

Addressing the Impact of Tobacco and Alcohol Use on Cancer-Related Health Outcomes

Convened March 17–18, 2025

Francis Amankwah, Michael Zierler,
and Sharyl Nass, *Rapporteurs*

National Cancer Policy Forum

Board on Health Care Services

Health and Medicine Division

Proceedings of a Workshop

NATIONAL ACADEMIES PRESS 500 Fifth Street, NW Washington, DC 20001

This activity was supported by Contract No. 75D30121D11240 (Task Order Nos. 75D30121F00002 and 75D30123F00024) and Contract No. 75N98024D00037 (Task Order No. 75N98025F00002) with the Centers for Disease Control and Prevention and the National Cancer Institute/National Institutes of Health, respectively, and by the American Association for Cancer Research; American Cancer Society; American College of Radiology; American Society of Clinical Oncology; Association of American Cancer Institutes; Association of Cancer Care Centers; Cancer Center at Illinois; Flatiron Health; Merck; National Comprehensive Cancer Network; Novartis Oncology; Oncology Nursing Society; Partners In Health; Patient Advocate Foundation; and Pfizer Inc. Any opinions, findings, conclusions, or recommendations expressed in this publication do not necessarily reflect the views of any organization or agency that provided support for the project.

International Standard Book Number-13: 978-0-309-60011-8
Digital Object Identifier: https://doi.org/10.17226/29264

This publication is available from the National Academies Press, 500 Fifth Street, NW, Keck 360, Washington, DC 20001; (800) 624–6242; https://nap.nationalacademies.org.

The manufacturer's authorized representative in the European Union for product safety is Authorised Rep Compliance Ltd., Ground Floor, 71 Lower Baggot Street, Dublin D02 P593 Ireland; www.arccompliance.com.

Printed in the United States of America.

Suggested citation: National Academies of Sciences, Engineering, and Medicine. 2025. *Addressing the impact of tobacco and alcohol use on cancer-related health outcomes: Proceedings of a workshop.* Washington, DC: National Academies Press. https://doi.org/10.17226/29264.

The **National Academy of Sciences** was established in 1863 by an Act of Congress, signed by President Lincoln, as a private, nongovernmental institution to advise the nation on issues related to science and technology. Members are elected by their peers for outstanding contributions to research. Dr. Marcia McNutt is president.

The **National Academy of Engineering** was established in 1964 under the charter of the National Academy of Sciences to bring the practices of engineering to advising the nation. Members are elected by their peers for extraordinary contributions to engineering. Dr. Tsu-Jae Liu is president.

The **National Academy of Medicine** (formerly the Institute of Medicine) was established in 1970 under the charter of the National Academy of Sciences to advise the nation on medical and health issues. Members are elected by their peers for distinguished contributions to medicine and health. Dr. Victor J. Dzau is president.

The three Academies work together as the **National Academies of Sciences, Engineering, and Medicine** to provide independent, objective analysis and advice to the nation and conduct other activities to solve complex problems and inform public policy decisions. The National Academies also encourage education and research, recognize outstanding contributions to knowledge, and increase public understanding in matters of science, engineering, and medicine.

Learn more about the National Academies of Sciences, Engineering, and Medicine at **www.nationalacademies.org**.

Consensus Study Reports published by the National Academies of Sciences, Engineering, and Medicine document the evidence-based consensus on the study's statement of task by an authoring committee of experts. Reports typically include findings, conclusions, and recommendations based on information gathered by the committee and the committee's deliberations. Each report has been subjected to a rigorous and independent peer-review process and it represents the position of the National Academies on the statement of task.

Proceedings published by the National Academies of Sciences, Engineering, and Medicine chronicle the presentations and discussions at a workshop, symposium, or other event convened by the National Academies. The statements and opinions contained in proceedings are those of the participants and are not endorsed by other participants, the planning committee, or the National Academies.

Rapid Expert Consultations published by the National Academies of Sciences, Engineering, and Medicine are authored by subject-matter experts on narrowly focused topics that can be supported by a body of evidence. The discussions contained in rapid expert consultations are considered those of the authors and do not contain policy recommendations. Rapid expert consultations are reviewed by the institution before release.

For information about other products and activities of the National Academies, please visit www.nationalacademies.org/about/whatwedo.

WORKSHOP PLANNING COMMITTEE

S. GAIL ECKHARDT (*Co-Chair*), Baylor College of Medicine
ROY S. HERBST (*Co-Chair*), Yale University; American Association for Cancer Research
GWEN DARIEN, Patient Advocate Foundation
SCARLETT LIN GOMEZ, University of California, San Francisco
CHANITA HUGHES-HALBERT, University of Southern California
FARHAD ISLAMI, American Cancer Society
ROY A. JENSEN, University of Kansas; Association of American Cancer Institutes
ELENA MARTÍNEZ, University of California San Diego
NIGAR NARGIS, American Cancer Society
LISA RICHARDSON, Centers for Disease Control and Prevention
DEIDRA ROACH, National Institute on Alcohol Abuse and Alcoholism
KATRINA TRIVERS, Centers for Disease Control and Prevention

Project Staff

ANNA ADLER, Research Associate (*from June 2025*)
TORRIE BROWN, Program Coordinator
MAKEDA HAUGHTON, Senior Program Assistant (*from December 2024*)
EMMA WICKLAND, Research Associate (*through May 2025*)
JULIE WILTSHIRE, Senior Finance Business Partner
JENNIFER ZHU, Associate Program Officer
FRANCIS AMANKWAH, Director, National Cancer Policy Forum
SHARYL NASS, Senior Director, Board on Health Care Services

NATIONAL CANCER POLICY FORUM

Forum Staff

ANNA ADLER, Research Associate
TORRIE BROWN, Program Coordinator
MAKEDA HAUGHTON, Senior Program Assistant
JULIE WILTSHIRE, Senior Finance Business Partner
JENNIFER ZHU, Associate Program Officer
FRANCIS AMANKWAH, Director, National Cancer Policy Forum
SHARYL NASS, Senior Director, Board on Health Care Services

Reviewers

This Proceedings of a Workshop was reviewed in draft form by individuals chosen for their diverse perspectives and technical expertise. The purpose of this independent review is to provide candid and critical comments that will assist the National Academies of Sciences, Engineering, and Medicine in making each published proceedings as sound as possible and to ensure that it meets the institutional standards for quality, objectivity, evidence, and responsiveness to the charge. The review comments and draft manuscript remain confidential to protect the integrity of the process.

We thank the following individuals for their review of this proceedings:

JENNIFER HAY, Memorial Sloan Kettering Cancer Center
KURT RIBISL, University of North Carolina Gillings School of Global Public Health

Although the reviewers listed above provided many constructive comments and suggestions, they were not asked to endorse the content of the proceedings, nor did they see the final draft before its release. The review of this proceedings was overseen by **PATRICIA GANZ,** University of California, Los Angeles. She was responsible for making certain that an independent examination of this proceedings was carried out in accordance with the standards of the National Academies and that all review comments were carefully considered. Responsibility for the final content rests entirely with the rapporteurs and the National Academies.

Acknowledgments

The National Cancer Policy Forum is grateful for the support of its many annual sponsors. Federal sponsors include the Centers for Disease Control and Prevention and National Cancer Institute/National Institutes of Health. Nonfederal sponsors include the American Association for Cancer Research, American Cancer Society, American College of Radiology, American Society of Clinical Oncology, Association of American Cancer Institutes, Association of Cancer Care Centers, Cancer Center at Illinois, Flatiron Health, Merck, National Comprehensive Cancer Network, Novartis Oncology, Oncology Nursing Society, Partners In Health, Patient Advocate Foundation, and Pfizer Inc.

The forum wishes to express its gratitude to the expert speakers whose presentations and discussions helped inform a deeper understanding of the effects of both tobacco and alcohol and their synergistic effects on cancer incidence and outcomes, education on the impacts of alcohol and tobacco, and the development of clinical guidelines for patients with cancer to mitigate the risks of alcohol and tobacco use. The forum also wishes to thank the members of the planning committee for their work in developing an excellent workshop agenda.

Contents

Boxes and Figure

BOXES

FIGURE

Acronyms and Abbreviations

ACS	American Cancer Society
AIAN	American Indian and Alaska Native
APHA	American Public Health Association
AUD	alcohol use disorder
DGA	Dietary Guidelines for Americans
FCTC	Framework Convention on Tobacco Control
FDA	U.S. Food and Drug Administration
GLP-1	glucagon-like peptide-1
IARC	International Agency for Research on Cancer
LEADS	Lung Cancer Education, Awareness, Detection, and Survivorship
NCI	National Cancer Institute
NIH	National Institutes of Health
WHO	World Health Organization

Proceedings of a Workshop

WORKSHOP OVERVIEW

The 1964 landmark report from the U.S. Surgeon General's Advisory Committee on Smoking and Health concluded that cigarette smoking led to an increased risk for lung cancer and chronic illness. The report recommended "appropriate remedial action" to reduce the health burdens from cigarette smoking in the United States (HHS, 1964). Congress responded rapidly by enacting laws that required health warnings on cigarette packs, banned cigarette advertising in broadcast media, and mandated reporting on the health consequences of smoking tobacco.[1,2]

Over the past 60 years, evidence for the link between cancer and tobacco use and between cancer and exposure to secondhand tobacco smoke has become undeniable, and the underlying physiological mechanisms have become clearer. Federal and state policy efforts and public health strategies have also coalesced, with the goal of reducing the health burdens from tobacco use (HHS, 2020a). However, use of tobacco products remains the leading modifiable risk factor for cancer incidence and death (Islami et al., 2024).

Evidence on the effects of alcohol consumption on health outcomes and cancer incidence has also increased in recent years. In 2025, the U.S. surgeon

---

[1] See Federal Cigarette Labeling and Advertising Act, https://www.ftc.gov/legal-library/browse/statutes/federal-cigarette-labeling-advertising-act (accessed June 20, 2025).

[2] See Public Health Cigarette Smoking Act of 1969, https://www.congress.gov/bill/91st-congress/house-bill/6543/text (accessed June 20, 2025).

general released an advisory that highlighted the link between alcohol use and cancer and called for measures to increase awareness of alcohol's contribution to cancer incidence and outcomes (HHS, 2025). Alcohol use is the third-ranked modifiable risk factor attributed to cancer morbidity and mortality (Islami et al., 2018). Data also show that individuals who smoke are more likely to consume alcohol and vice versa (van Amsterdam and van den Brink, 2023).

To examine the state of the science on the links between tobacco use and alcohol consumption and cancer incidence and outcomes as well as opportunities to reduce tobacco and alcohol use to lower cancer risk and improve health outcomes, the National Cancer Policy Forum of the National Academies of Sciences, Engineering, and Medicine (the National Academies) hosted a workshop on March 17 and 18, 2025. The workshop was held in collaboration with the National Academies Forum on Mental Health and Substance Use Disorders. Participants brought expertise in the behavioral, basic, and clinical sciences; patient advocacy; community engagement; public health; and health economics.

This Proceedings of a Workshop summarizes the presentations and discussions. The comments from individual participants are discussed throughout the proceedings and summarized in Boxes 1 (observations on the effects of alcohol and tobacco use on cancer-related health outcomes) and 2 (suggestions to advance progress in reducing tobacco and alcohol use to lower cancer risk and improve health outcomes). Appendixes A and B include the Statement of Task and agenda, respectively. Speaker presentations and the webcast are archived online.[3]

OVERVIEW OF RESEARCH ON THE IMPACT OF TOBACCO AND ALCOHOL USE ON CANCER-RELATED HEALTH OUTCOMES

A substantial proportion of U.S. cancer cases and deaths is attributable to modifiable risk factors. Many participants discussed the state of research on tobacco use and alcohol consumption as modifiable risk factors[4] for cancer and related health outcomes, differences in outcomes among U.S. populations, risk

---

[3] See workshop website, https://www.nationalacademies.org/event/43170_03-2025_addressing-the-impact-of-tobacco-and-alcohol-use-on-cancer-related-health-outcomes-a-workshop (accessed March 28, 2025).

[4] These are behaviors and exposures that can raise or lower a person's risk of cancer. See https://cancercontrol.cancer.gov/research-emphasis/future-directions/modifiable-risk-factors (accessed April 21, 2025).

implications for people who use both tobacco and alcohol, and awareness of the associations between tobacco use, alcohol use, and cancer.

Tobacco Use and Cancer-Related Health Outcomes

Farhad Islami from the American Cancer Society (ACS) said that tobacco use and alcohol consumption are the first and third leading modifiable risk factors for cancer cases and deaths in the United States, respectively (Islami et al., 2018, 2024). In 2019, cigarette smoking contributed to 19 percent of cancer cases and nearly 29 percent of cancer-related deaths (Islami et al., 2024). Neal Freedman from the National Institutes of Health (NIH) stressed the profound impact that cigarette smoking has on cancer risk. He also pointed out the growing popularity of other heated and smokeless tobacco products. According to the World Health Organization (WHO), more than 1.2 billion people around the world use tobacco, and people who smoke lose 5–10 years of life on average compared to the median lifespan of 85 years among people who never smoked (Inoue-Choi et al., 2019). Based on data analyzed from the 2019–2022 National Health Interview Surveys, approximately one in five U.S. adults currently use some type of tobacco product.[5] People who smoke cigarettes comprised 59 percent of those users, and most of the tobacco-related diseases and deaths are linked to cigarette smoking (CDC, 2024).

Freedman, David Berrigan from NIH, Brian King[6] from the U.S. Food and Drug Administration (FDA), and several other participants pointed out that significant progress has been made since the surgeon general's 1964 report on smoking and health. Tobacco control measures have led to a steady decline in cigarette use from 1964 through present (see Figure 1). These public health measures—education, bans on advertising tobacco products, financial disincentives, litigation, and raising the minimum purchase age—have directly led to a drop in the rates of cancer incidence and mortality, especially for lung cancer. Nonetheless, much can still be done to further reduce the burden of disease from use of cigarettes and other tobacco products. Furthermore, progress in reducing tobacco use has not occurred evenly nationwide. This variation is due in part to differences in state and local policies (CDC, 2025; Chakraborty et al., 2025; Patel et al., 2023). For example, Freedman and Islami said that the prevalence of smoking is greatest in parts of the South, Appalachia, Alaska, and Nevada, which also experience the highest rates of cancer deaths attributable to smoking (Lortet-Tieulent et al., 2016).

---

[5] See Tobacco Product Use Among Adults—United States, 2022, https://www.cdc.gov/tobacco/media/pdfs/2024/09/cdc-osh-ncis-data-report-508.pdf (accessed April 22, 2025).

[6] Dr. King is currently working at the Campaign for Tobacco-Free Kids.

BOX 1
Observations from Individual Workshop Participants on the Effects of Tobacco and Alcohol Use on Cancer-Related Health Outcomes

Impact of Tobacco and Alcohol Use on Cancer Risk

- Tobacco and alcohol are the first and third leading modifiable risk factors for cancer cases and deaths in the United States, respectively. (Islami)
- Less than half the U.S. adult population is aware that alcohol is a modifiable risk factor for cancer and that there are cancer sites with established increased risk associated with alcohol. (Freudenheim, Hay, Klein)
- Nearly one-quarter of the global cancer burden is linked to tobacco and alcohol use, and many people, including youth and young adults, co-use both substances. (Barrington-Trimis, Faseru, Justice, Rumgay)
- Early prevention strategies are critical to reducing the health burdens from tobacco because about 90 percent of people who smoke began before the age of 18 and nearly all smokers (around 99 percent) started before the age of 26. (King, Ling)
- Smoking by patients diagnosed with cancer and cancer survivors causes adverse health outcomes including increased overall mortality, cancer-related mortality, risk for second primary cancer, and associations with increased toxicity from cancer treatment. (Warren)
- Smoking cessation after a cancer diagnosis has the potential to improve cancer treatment outcomes and improve overall survival, with optimal benefits achieved by quitting smoking within 6 months following a cancer diagnosis. (Warren)

Communication about Tobacco and Alcohol as Modifiable Risk Factors

- When discussing tobacco use with Indigenous communities, it is important to distinguish between commercial and traditional tobacco; the latter is considered sacred and used as medicine, gifts, and offerings. (Buffalo)
- The consumption of alcohol is embedded in our society and intertwined with meals and festivities, making the messaging about alcohol-linked cancer risk challenging. (Berrigan, Eck, Fong)

- Public health messaging about alcohol-related cancer risk is a work in progress and cannot take the same approach as that for tobacco-related cancer risks. (Fong, Klein)
- Addressing labeling and dietary guidelines involves both complex science and some intensely competing interests and perspectives. (Berrigan)

Cessation Measures

- Quitlines have shown effectiveness for tobacco cessation, via translation of behavioral research into public health services. (King, Toll, Zhu)
- Tobacco cessation resources are not equitably accessible across populations. (Cartujano-Barrera, Greene-Moton, Okuyemi)
- Pharmaceutical interventions, like nicotine replacement therapy and receptor agonists (e.g., varenicline and semaglutide), could be promising cessation treatment for alcohol/tobacco co-use. (Faseru, Toll)
- Smoking cessation approaches after a cancer diagnosis have not kept pace with the innovations in other cancer treatments. (Warren)

Tobacco and Alcohol Policies

- Taxation and, to a lesser extent, minimum pricing regulations raise the prices of tobacco and alcohol products, and consumers react to price by decreasing consumption, making these very effective population-level tactics for reducing use, especially in combination with bans on promotions and discounts at the point of sale. (Drope, Fong, Nargis, Ribisl)
- Counter-marketing interventions that target specific populations have been successful at reducing the prevalence of smoking and heavy/binge drinking. (Fong, Ling)
- Marketing efforts by the tobacco and alcohol industries run counter to the public health measures that encourage people to quit. (Eck, Fong, Ling, Okuyemi)

NOTE: This list is the rapporteurs' synopsis of observations made by one or more individual speakers as identified. These statements have not been endorsed or verified by the National Academies of Sciences, Engineering, and Medicine. They are not intended to reflect a consensus among workshop participants.

BOX 2
Suggestions from Individual Workshop Participants to Lower Cancer Risk and Improve Health Outcomes by Reducing Tobacco and Alcohol Use

Improving Public Health Messaging

- Deliver the message about the link between alcohol and cancer risk with empathy, support, and hope and without blame or shame. (Carter-Bawa, Darien, Hay, Okuyemi)
- Consider current social norms when crafting public health messaging about the cancer-related risk of alcohol consumption. (Fong)
- Craft messaging that is based on scientific evidence and acknowledges that susceptibility varies among individuals based on factors like age and health status when discussing the effects of alcohol consumption. (Berrigan, Hay, Justice, Westmaas)
- Increase public awareness of the link between alcohol and cancer, which could strengthen public support for measures to reduce alcohol consumption. (Berrigan, Hay, Justice, Klein)
- Help people trying to quit tobacco or alcohol through repeated exposure to cessation advice and support. (Westmaas, Zhu)
- Formulate a community-driven public health communication strategy about the cancer-related risks of tobacco and alcohol use that includes counter-advertising and appeals to shared values, like the importance of family and community and protecting our youth. (Eck, Fong, Hay, Ling)

Enhancing Policy Efforts

- Work within communities and with policy makers to develop and improve evidence-based tobacco and alcohol policies that reflect the impacts on individuals and communities. (Buffalo, Cartujano-Barrera, Evers, Jordan)
- Improve the enforcement of policies restricting the sale of tobacco and alcohol. (Barrington-Trimis, Leventhal, Ribisl)
- Increase funds to support tobacco cessation efforts and other public health campaigns through excise taxes and legal settlements. (Okuyemi, Ribisl)

Exploring Areas for Additional Research

- Broaden research on how e-cigarettes and other emerging tobacco products are related to cancer. (Freedman, Hecht, Ling, Toll)
- Expand research on alcohol and cancer in understudied areas, including the effects of heavy episodic drinking, effects of drinking

pattern, drinking across the life-span, drinking following a cancer diagnosis, and alcohol-related links to specific cancers. (Calonge, Freudenheim, Nargis)

- Further investigate the effects of tobacco and alcohol co-use on cancer outcomes, including identification of optimal cancer treatment strategies among patients with a former or current smoking status. (Berrigan, Justice, Ling, Warren, Zhou)
- Extend research to assess the crossover effects that alcohol and tobacco policies have on behavioral changes in the use of each product and co-use of both products. (King, Ling)
- Expand research on cessation medications that could help people who co-use tobacco with alcohol or cannabis. (Barrington-Trimis, Faseru, Toll)
- Leverage community-based participatory research to improve the study and practice of prevention, cessation, and harm reduction efforts. (Cartujano-Barrera, Greene-Moton, Jordan, Winn)
- Create more opportunities for collaborative research between scientists and public health officials who work on tobacco or alcohol. (Leventhal, Ling, Nargis)
- Conduct additional research to quantitate optimal alcohol tax rates based on the health costs of alcohol consumption; identify heterogeneity in price responsiveness by population characteristics and baseline alcohol consumption patterns; and measure the economic impact of alcohol taxation to counteract alcohol industry arguments against tax increases. (Drope, Nargis)

Advancing Potential Opportunities to Support Cessation

- Translate the success of tobacco cessation quitlines to cessation and reduction strategies for alcohol and cannabis by focusing on replicable elements, such as identifying and avoiding triggers; counseling on coping and avoidance mechanisms; and providing motivation, encouragement, and support throughout the journey. (Westmaas, Zhu)
- Collaborate with medical accrediting, policy, and guideline organizations to make smoking cessation a standard of cancer care to improve cancer treatment rather than focusing on it only as a form of prevention. (Warren)

NOTE: This list is the rapporteurs' synopsis of suggestions made by one or more individual speakers as identified. These statements have not been endorsed or verified by the National Academies of Sciences, Engineering, and Medicine. They are not intended to reflect a consensus among workshop participants.

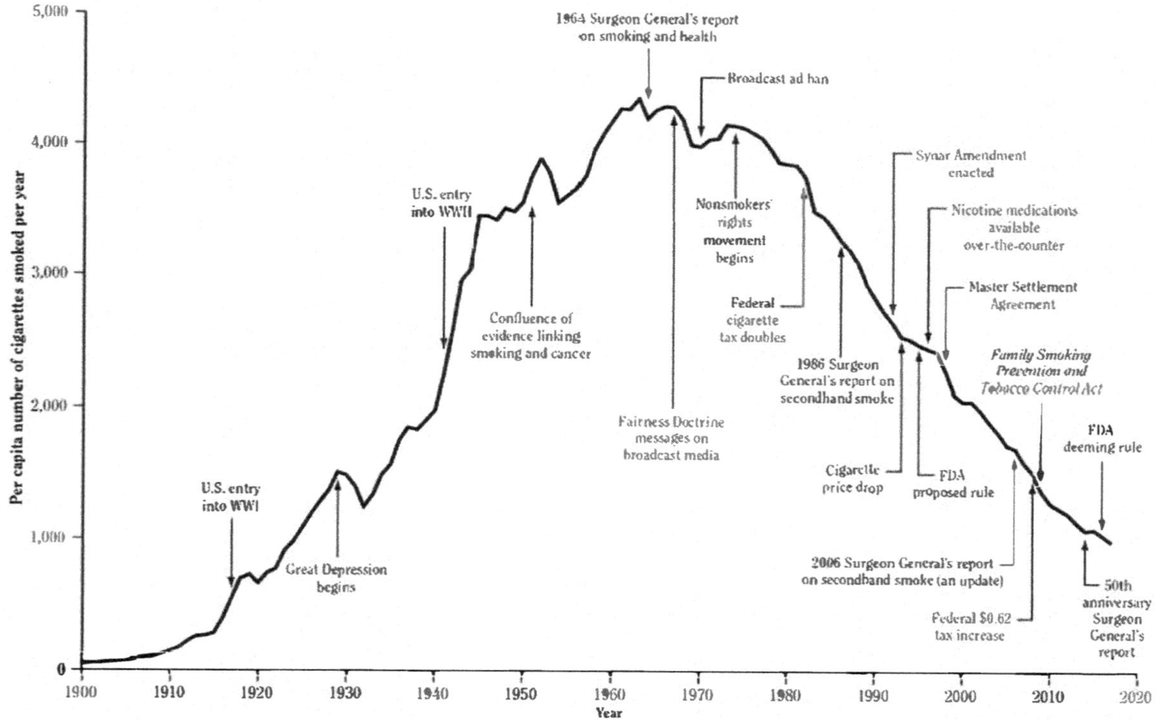

FIGURE 1 U.S. cigarette consumption, 1900–2020.
SOURCES: Freedman, Hay, and Ribisl Presentations, March 17, 2025; HHS, 2020a, derived from Warner and Goldenhar, 1985, with permission from Massachusetts Medical Society © 1985, as cited in HHS, 2014.

Alcohol Use and Cancer-Related Health Outcomes

According to the 2025 surgeon general's advisory on alcohol and cancer risk, alcohol contributes to nearly 100,000 cancer cases and about 20,000 cancer deaths in the United States each year. Berrigan said that the evidence linking alcohol to cancer has been established using the same types of rigorous evidence and review as for tobacco. Harriet Rumgay from the International Agency for Research on Cancer (IARC) stressed that, as with tobacco products, the IARC has classified alcohol as a Group I carcinogen.[7]

Nearly one-quarter of the global cancer burden is due to tobacco and alcohol use (Reitsma et al., 2021; Rumgay et al., 2021b, 2024). The mechanisms by which alcohol increases the risk of cancer include DNA damage due to the breakdown of alcohol into acetaldehyde in the body; oxidative stress that damages DNA, triggers abnormal cell functioning, and increases inflammation; altered levels of several hormones; and alcohol dissolving other carcinogens, making them more easily absorbed into the body (Rumgay et al., 2021a).

The Dietary Guidelines for Americans (DGA) recommends limiting the intake of alcohol to two drinks per day for men and one drink per day for women.[8,9] This is considered moderate consumption. Jo Freudenheim from the University at Buffalo defined heavy consumption as exceeding these recommendations. Freudenheim said that there is established evidence for multiple sites in the body, including the esophagus, liver, breast, head and neck (i.e., oral cavity, pharynx, and larynx), and colorectum, that alcohol consumption increases risk (HHS, 2025; NCI and WHO, 2016). Further, there is sufficient evidence that reduction in alcohol consumption is associated with decreased risk for oral and squamous cell esophageal cancer as well as limited evidence for reduced risk for laryngeal, colorectal, and breast cancers (Gapstur et al., 2023). Rumgay said that the global burden of cancer attributable to drinking alcohol was about 741,000 cases, or around 4 percent of all cancer cases, in 2020, and esophageal, liver, and breast cancers accounted for 60 percent of that (Rumgay et al., 2021a). She pointed out that about half of global cancer cases due to alcohol were in people whose consumption is in the heavy drinking category (>60 grams alcohol per day); moderate (<20 grams per day) and

---

[7] See IARC Monographs on the Identification of Carcinogenic Hazards to Humans: https://monographs.iarc.who.int/agents-classified-by-the-iarc/ (accessed June 20, 2025).

[8] See Dietary Guidelines for Americans 2020–2025, https://www.dietaryguidelines.gov/sites/default/files/2021-03/Dietary_Guidelines_for_Americans-2020-2025.pdf (accessed April 22, 2025).

[9] The DGA defines a drink equivalent as 14 grams (0.6 fluid ounces) of pure alcohol. One drink contains the amount of alcohol in a drink equivalent, such as 12 fluid ounces of regular beer (5 percent alcohol), 5 fluid ounces of wine (12 percent alcohol), or 1.5 fluid ounces of 80 proof distilled spirits (40 percent alcohol).

risky (20–60 grams per day) drinking made up the other half (Rumgay et al., 2021a). Freudenheim also noted a linear dose response for breast cancer risk associated with alcohol consumption, adding that there is no evidence of a minimum threshold, and a small amount of alcohol consumption results in a small increase in cancer risk.

Despite multiple risk factors for alcohol use disorder (AUD), a medical condition marked by difficulty controlling use, Hang Zhou from Yale School of Medicine highlighted the significant role of genetics.[10] Zhou explained that in a genome-wide association study of more than 1 million people, researchers identified 110 risk variants associated with AUD (Zhou et al., 2023a). Using Mendelian randomization,[11] Zhou and colleagues analyzed the causal impacts of AUD on various cancers (Zhou and Vasiliou, 2022; Zhou et al., 2023b). With 74 single-nucleotide polymorphisms as the instrumental variables, the study found suggestive positive effects of AUD on oral cancers.

Freudenheim pointed out some remaining research gaps, including the need for more data on the effects of heavy episodic drinking and of drinking pattern on cancer risk (e.g., drinking 1 day a week but having six or seven drinks in that single sitting); longitudinal data on people who drink heavily as teenagers and young adults but then later reduce their consumption; and the effects of alcohol on people who have received a cancer diagnosis, including alcohol's impact on treatment outcomes, the formation of second primary tumors, and cancer prognosis more broadly. She concluded by noting that these risks have been more thoroughly studied for tobacco than for alcohol.

Ned Calonge from the Colorado School of Public Health summarized the parts of the National Academies consensus report, *Review of Evidence on Alcohol and Health*, that reviewed the scientific evidence on the relationship between alcohol consumption and health outcomes (NASEM, 2025). Calonge said that the report focused on the relationship between moderate alcohol consumption as defined by the DGA[12] and eight specific health outcomes, including cardiovascular disease, all-cause mortality, and certain types of cancer, including breast and colorectal. Calonge said that the committee excluded studies in which former drinkers and never drinkers were combined, to avoid

---

[10] The National Institute on Alcohol Abuse and Alcoholism says that the hereditability of AUD is approximately 60 percent. See https://www.niaaa.nih.gov/publications/brochures-and-fact-sheets/understanding-alcohol-use-disorder (accessed May 12, 2025).

[11] Mendelian randomization studies use genetic variation associated with modifiable exposures (potential risk factors) to assess their possible causal relationship with the related health outcomes, aiming to reduce potential bias from confounding and reverse causation.

[12] According to the 2020–2025 DGA, moderate alcohol consumption is two drinks or fewer per day for men and one drink or fewer per day for women, where a drink is defined as containing 14 grams of alcohol.

introducing "abstainer bias," because former drinkers can include people who quit for health reasons and therefore cause an overestimation of the potential benefits of moderate drinking, he said. The committee looked at studies that considered the cancer-related impacts of alcohol on breast, oral, pharyngeal, and colorectal cancers.

Based on a systematic review, the committee determined that women who consume moderate amounts of alcohol have approximately a 10 percent increased risk of developing breast cancer compared to never drinkers. The committee performed two additional meta-analyses. It found that for each increase of 0.7–1.0 drinks per day, there was a 5 percent increase in risk of breast cancer. Among women with moderate intakes, those with higher moderate consumption had increased risk compared to those with lower moderate consumption, Calonge said.

Regarding colorectal cancer, Calonge said that the number of usable studies was limited, so the evidence failed to meet statistical significance, leading the committee to conclude that no conclusions could be drawn about the association between moderate alcohol consumption and the risk compared with never drinkers. Calonge said that to determine whether there is an association, additional research with larger cohort sizes would be valuable.

Calonge identified a number of methodological challenges and areas for future research. He asked, "Is there a difference between a drink per day for a week versus seven drinks in 1 day in a week? Are there mitigating or augmenting effects of eating while drinking alcohol?" He added that self-reporting about alcohol use often leads to underreporting. He suggested that it would be essential for studies to include information about age; sex; genetic ancestry; socioeconomic status; education; diet; and, for breast cancer, menopausal status, so that confounders, effect modifiers, and residual confounding can be accounted for. He added that to use Mendelian randomization for investigating the health impacts of moderate alcohol use, basic science needs to identify the set of genes that adequately captures differences in alcohol intake.

Synergistic Effects of Alcohol and Tobacco Use on Cancer-Related Health Outcomes

Berrigan said that synergistic increases in risk of certain cancers from co-use of alcohol and tobacco have been documented. Stephen Hecht from the University of Minnesota said that this is especially evident for head and neck cancer. Freudenheim and Berrigan both pointed out that heavy drinkers who also smoke increase their risk of head and neck cancers by 5–14 times compared to people who never smoke or drink. Hecht explained that alcohol enhances the formation of adducts between DNA and tobacco carcinogens in oral cells, though the mechanisms are not fully understood (Hashibe et al., 2009). Hecht noted an ongoing study to better understand the synergistic health impacts of co-using alcohol and tobacco by comparing three groups: people who never smoke or drink (or drink only lightly), people who smoke but never drink (or drink lightly), and people who smoke and are moderate to heavy drinkers. Investigators isolate the oral cell DNA from the participants and identify DNA adducts using a combination of liquid chromatography and tandem mass spectrometry. He said that although the mechanisms by which alcohol and tobacco carcinogens interact to increase cancer risk have not been fully elucidated, potential theories include that alcohol may increase the permeability of the oral mucosa to the tobacco carcinogens, alcohol may inhibit carcinogen detoxification enzymes, and tobacco smoke may alter the formation of acetaldehyde from alcohol by the oral microbiome (IARC, 2012; Stornetta et al., 2018). Hecht added that there is evidence that vaping causes DNA damage in the oral mucosa; however, research is necessary to assess whether alcohol enhances DNA damage in co-users of alcohol (Stornetta et al., 2018).

Zhou and his colleagues used multivariable Mendelian randomization to assess an independent genetic relationship between AUD and oral cancer, controlling for alcohol consumption and tobacco smoking traits. Their results indicated direct effects of AUD and smoking status (current smoker vs. former smoker) on oral cancer (Zhou et al., 2023b). Zhou urged researchers to be cautious when interpreting these results because they are preliminary and also focused on effects of genetic liability to a disease, rather than an observation of the disease per se, and he urged further research on these synergistic genetic effects.

Awareness of Tobacco- and Alcohol-Related Cancer Risk

Berrigan noted the greater awareness of the link between tobacco and cancer than the link between alcohol and cancer among U.S. adults. He highlighted that the awareness of the link between tobacco and cancer increased from 40 percent in 1965 to about 90 percent by 2019 (AICR, 2020; HHS, 2014).

Jennifer Hay from Memorial Sloan Kettering Cancer Center and William Klein from NIH also stressed that the awareness of the cancer harms of alcohol use is relatively low. According to one study based on data collected from a nationally representative sample, 18 percent of adults believe that alcohol has no effect; more than half do not know it has any connection with cancer; and about 10 percent believe that wine, in particular, decreases the risk of cancer (Seidenberg et al., 2023). Klein said that one reason most people are not aware of the link between alcohol and cancer is that clinicians do not routinely share this information with patients (Wiseman et al., 2022). Klein said that increasing public awareness of this link may lead to greater public support for stronger policies that aim to reduce alcohol use and accessibility

(Seidenberg et al., 2022). He noted the positive correlation between people being aware of the link and support for alcohol policy measures. Hay agreed, stating that creating awareness is a critical early step in addressing this public health problem, in much the same way that the 1964 surgeon general's report was "that inflection point for tobacco."

Berrigan pointed out that co-use of tobacco and alcohol is significant among people who drink more than the U.S. guidelines, so it is important to address in those populations, because the risk factors can be synergistic and the approaches for educating, counseling, and helping people to quit may differ somewhat from those for people who use only alcohol or tobacco. He encouraged researchers to think about the uses of their results and how they might contribute more directly to the evidence needed for changing specific policies.

CURRENT POLICY STRATEGIES TO REDUCE TOBACCO AND ALCOHOL USE

Efforts to reduce the public health burden of tobacco products in the United States have been expansive and ongoing for decades (HHS, 2020a). Similar efforts to reduce alcohol consumption have been less comprehensive, more recent, and initially focused on injuries and deaths from drunk driving (Blanchette et al., 2020).

Many participants provided an overview of policy strategies that have helped to reduce tobacco use and encouraged a reduction in alcohol use. Several highlighted the similarities and differences among the strategies aimed at reducing tobacco versus alcohol use and lessons from the two fields that can be applied to lower cancer risk and improve health outcomes.

King said that tobacco control efforts serve as an example of effectively translating science into public health practices, stressing that effective control efforts span individual, health system, and population levels (see Box 3). He noted the useful lessons from work in the tobacco control field over the past decades. Mark Evers from the University of Kentucky Markey Cancer Center discussed the challenges and successes that Kentucky has had in addressing its tobacco-related cancer burden (see Box 4).

Taxes and Pricing Policies

Jeffrey Drope from the Johns Hopkins Bloomberg School of Public Health said that the price of inelastic goods, like tobacco products and alcoholic beverages, is a very important factor in consumer decision making.[13]

[13] Price inelastic goods are items that do not greatly change in demand when prices fluctuate. This is different from perfectly inelastic, in which consumer demand does not change at all when prices fluctuate.

BOX 3
A Perspective on Why Tobacco Control Efforts Have Been Effective

King identified three overarching approaches that have been used successfully in reducing tobacco-related disease and death: prevention, cessation, and harm reduction. He said that prevention is critical because about 90 percent of people who smoke began before the age of 18, and nearly all smokers (around 99 percent) start smoking before the age of 26 (HHS, 2014). He added that engaging young people in the message that they do not need to use tobacco products greatly reduces the health burden. Cessation programs are a second part of the approach, King said. These include population-level interventions and individual treatment regimens, such as quitlines, text messages, and medications. Third, King said, is harm reduction, especially as the tobacco product landscape has diversified, with people switching from smoking tobacco to other lower-risk products.

King said that effective cancer control efforts require comprehensive strategies at the individual, health system, and population levels (Califf and King, 2023). He identified four key components that have helped to drive the success of the overarching approaches. He said the first is population-based efforts, including policies that increased tobacco prices, created smoke-free settings, raised the minimum age of sale to 21 years, restricted advertising and promotions, and facilitated mass-reach health communication campaigns and advice from clinicians and other health care professionals. King added that it is essential to identify novel strategies through continued research and innovation. Federal regulation has been a significant bulwark in supporting population-based strategies, King added. For example, the 2009 Family Smoking Prevention and Tobacco Control Act[a] implemented a wide range of tobacco controls, such as enabling the FDA Center for Tobacco Products to implement standards for tobacco products to protect public health.

The second component King discussed is the complementary efforts across the federal, state, and local levels of government. By working in overlapping ways, branches of FDA and state and local authorities have been able to apply significant control over the marketing, sale, and use of tobacco products. King also said that regulatory efforts often percolate upward once a local municipality makes a change. For example, he said, Needham, Massachusetts, was the first U.S. locality to raise the tobacco sales age to 21 years. A few years later, other cities and states followed suit, and Congress made it a federal law in 2019.[b]

The third component is data-driven methods. King said that policy changes and substance control efforts need to be built on a foundation of solid scientific evidence. King also pointed out that while data are essential for developing policy, they are also critical in shaping how policies are implemented, messaging is carried out, and public health efforts are evaluated and revised.

King said that the fourth component is the ability for public health efforts to be nimble and adaptable as the market evolves. He stressed that it is essential for public health to remain flexible to be able to revise messaging, strategies, and treatments as the evidence grows and society changes. For example, King said, earlier mass-reach campaigns targeting youth used antismoking ads on television. But in recent times, because tobacco products have diversified and youth spend far more time on the Internet than watching television, outreach is now in digital spaces and focuses on vaping and smokeless tobacco products. "We do not have to reinvent the wheel. It's making sure that we apply our standard, our foundation of science, and then use that in a way that's going to be impactful, but be mindful that things change," he concluded.

---

[a] See https://www.fda.gov/tobacco-products/rules-regulations-and-guidance-related-tobacco-products/family-smoking-prevention-and-tobacco-control-act-table-contents (accessed June 23, 2025).

[b] See https://www.congress.gov/bill/116th-congress/house-bill/2411/text (accessed June 23, 2025).

People react to both the absolute price and any price changes that occur for inelastic goods that are not perfectly inelastic. Thus, if taxes on alcohol and tobacco are increased, retail prices rise, people buy less, and consumption decreases. Related to price is the concept of affordability, which factors in people's income along with the price of goods. Drope said that alcoholic beverages in the United States are generally both inexpensive and affordable, adding that raising excise taxes could lead producers to raise prices to maintain their profits.

Drope explained that for alcohol, the price elasticity is about -0.5: if the price increases by 10 percent, consumption decreases by 5 percent (Guindon et al., 2022). Thus, raising taxes drives a decline in consumption due to price increases, but the increased revenue from higher taxes typically exceeds the loss of revenue from that decline. Drope suggested that the extra revenue can be earmarked for public health education efforts and harm reduction and cessation programs. Similarly, when prices rise on cigarettes, consumption declines. For example, a 10 percent price increase per pack leads to a 2.5–5 percent reduction in consumption (NCI and WHO, 2016).

Health Warning Labels on Product Packaging

Geoffrey T. Fong from University of Waterloo and Ontario Institute for Cancer Research said that Article 11 of the WHO Framework Convention on Tobacco Control (FCTC) calls on its parties[14] to implement policies and effective measures to ensure that packaging and labeling of tobacco products do not mislead people to conclude that these are safe to be consumed and that tobacco packaging carries health warnings that describe the harmful effects of use.[15] Health warnings on cigarette packs range from text-only labels on the side to a full suite of graphics and text that warn about the dangers of smoking and provide encouragement and information about quitting. Fong said that packaging health warning labels have been shown to be effective at increasing quit rates and reducing consumption (Brewer et al., 2016; Noar et al., 2016). The use of a variety of warning labels increases their effectiveness at reducing cigarette consumption and increasing the rate of quit attempts (Green et al., 2019). Some evidence suggests that tobacco warnings with pictures may be more effective than text-only messages at communicating health risk (Fong et al., 2009).

Kurt Ribisl from the University of North Carolina Gillings School of Global Public Health added that pictorial health warning labels on tobacco products are a cost-effective policy to promote awareness of smoking-related

[14] The United States is not a party to the WHO FCTC.

[15] See WHO FCTC, https://fctc.who.int/ (accessed June 20, 2025).

harms and smoking cessation because customers are exposed to the warning at the point of sale and every time they use the product; they are used by many countries and have withstood legal and political challenges. He also said they can improve health equity because people with low literacy can understand the warnings.

Warning labels on alcoholic beverages do not warn about the risk of cancer, but Berrigan said that the surgeon general's advisory on this risk has motivated some state legislatures to consider updating these labels. In addition, he said, the labels need to be larger, more prominent, and modified to be more effective at conveying the health risks. Berrigan added that addressing labeling and dietary guidelines for how much alcohol is okay involves both complex science and some intensely competing interests and perspectives, making this a classic public health problem. Fong noted that the cultural differences and social norms around how tobacco and alcohol are viewed may reduce the effectiveness of highly graphic warning labels on alcoholic beverages. Thus, different tools and approaches to educating people about the alcohol-related cancer risks may be needed.

Excise Taxes, Minimum Price Policies, and Marketing Restrictions

Ribisl noted that income and smoking prevalence are inversely related. For this reason, tobacco companies use price promotions at the point of sale that are geared to specific audiences. To counter these promotions, changes that raise the cost of tobacco products and prohibit discounting can potentially reduce consumption and increase quit rates, especially among lower-income groups. Ribisl said that it would be essential to have a multipronged policy approach to reduce consumption at all socioeconomic levels, including an increase in excise taxes,[16] minimum pricing requirements, and a ban on pricing promotions. In combination, these three policy changes would have numerous beneficial effects, including reducing health inequities, reducing smoking prevalence overall, and raising revenue for governments that could fund smoking cessation programs (Ribisl et al., 2022). He noted that establishing a minimum price on tobacco products reduces tobacco consumption disparities among socioeconomic groups more effectively than does increasing excise taxes alone (Golden et al., 2016).

To limit the use of tobacco flavorings as a marketing tool, eight states have passed bans or restrictions.[17] However, the data indicate that bans on flavored

---

[16] Unlike a general sales tax that applies to most retail purchases, excise taxes are levied only on a special class of items or activities.

[17] Based on data from the Public Health Law Center as of July 2024; provided by Dr. Barrington-Trimis, March 17, 2025.

BOX 4
Lessons from a State with High Smoking Prevalence

Evers said that Kentucky has the highest U.S. incidence and mortality rates of lung cancer (Rodriguez et al., 2018). This can be attributed, he said, to a combination of risk factors: a high poverty rate—7 percent of the population, including approximately 42 percent of the 120 counties that experience persistent poverty[a]—high rates of smoking and obesity, and low education levels. Evers said that reducing the state's cancer burden meant developing strategies to address all of these contributing factors. The Markey Cancer Center developed a series of strategies to address the significant impact of smoking on lung cancer. Such strategies have included implementing tobacco control efforts, educating health care professionals about routinely assessing a patient's smoking status and having empathic discussions with patients about the health impacts, developing smoking cessation programs, and expanding lung cancer screening efforts. The goal, Evers said, was to address smoking across the lung cancer continuum. Part of the strategy is to offer free cessation assistance to everyone with a cancer diagnosis who reported using tobacco in the previous month. In the first year of the program, tobacco use screening rates went from 63 percent to 92 percent among this patient population (Burris et al., 2022). The Lung Cancer Education, Awareness, Detection, and Survivorship (LEADS) Collaborative[b] provided continuing education to about 2,900 health care professionals focused on improving early detection of lung cancer and patient quality of care. Lung cancer was being undertreated in Kentucky, and LEADS was designed to reverse that by educating the health care workforce about the latest in diagnosis and treatment methods and efforts to increase smoking cessation. LEADS had two additional complementary components, said Evers: preventing and detecting lung cancer and improving survivorship care. Its success led to efforts to export the program to Mississippi and Nevada, which also have high lung cancer rates.[c]

Evers noted that although improved cancer treatments are increasing survival, many cancer survivors are not getting the care needed to support their mental health and quality of life. The Markey Cancer Center developed and implemented a "hope-based intervention" that was delivered to patients during cancer treatment through in-person sessions and telephone calls (McLouth et al., 2024).[d] It also had success in influencing statewide policy initiatives, including municipal smoke-free ordinances and the establishment of a lung cancer screening and prevention program within the state's Department of Public Health. All of these efforts, Evers said, have led to measurable improvements in reducing the state's lung cancer burden.[e] Kentucky is now the number two state in lung cancer screening rates; cancers are being detected earlier, resulting in declines in late-stage lung cancer incidence that outpace the national average. Evers emphasized that the success of these programs was only possible because community members were engaged in the decision-making process.

---

[a] An area is considered in persistent poverty if it had a poverty rate of 20.0 percent or higher during the three-decade period from 1989 to 2015–2019. See https://www.census.gov/library/stories/2023/05/persistent-poverty-areas-with-long-term-high-poverty.html (accessed May 19, 2025).

[b] For more information on the LEADS Collaborative, see https://www.kcp.uky.edu/partnerships/kentuckyleads.php (accessed June 20, 2025).

[c] A $6.8 million grant will allow the University of Kentucky and University of Colorado to expand their successful QUILS (Quality Implementation of Lung Cancer Screening) program, which has improved screening rates in Kentucky, to Mississippi and Nevada to address high lung cancer burdens and health disparities. See https://research.uky.edu/news/markey-researchers-awarded-68-million-help-others-replicate-kentuckys-lung-cancer-screening (accessed June 20, 2025).

[d] A hope-based intervention aims to increase patients' sense of hope by helping them reduce cancer-related goal interference, improve emotional outcomes, and support pursuit of meaningful goals (McLouth et al., 2024).

[e] State of Lung Cancer 2024 Report. See https://www.lung.org/getmedia/12020193-7fb3-46b8-8d78-0e5d9cd8f93c/SOLC-2024.pdf (accessed July 3, 2025).

tobacco products without suitable enforcement are ineffective (Chaffee et al., 2025).

Fong pointed out that bans on tobacco advertising, promotion, and sponsorship have also been effective in reducing smoking prevalence and initiation and increasing cessation rates (Saad et al., 2025). However, for alcohol, specific approaches and implementation strategies will be shaped by the public's perceptions, which differ significantly from those of tobacco use.

MESSAGING AND MARKETING OF TOBACCO AND ALCOHOL PRODUCTS

Many participants discussed the tension between marketing and public health messaging regarding tobacco and alcohol use.

Messaging and Marketing Tactics by the Tobacco and Alcohol Industries

Raimee Eck from the Johns Hopkins Bloomberg School of Public Health noted a huge difference in the messaging from industries like alcohol or tobacco versus the public health community. Eck added that the industries link their products and using them to a variety of shared values, such as freedom, sportsmanship, individualism, and patriotism. Public health messaging, on the other hand, is often heavy with data and negative framing that lose the audience. She said that young people who own alcohol-branded merchandise are more likely to start drinking and binge drinking (Jernigan et al., 2017). Increased exposure to alcohol advertising and marketing is positively correlated with young people starting to drink. Furthermore, Eck noted that the brands that spend more on youth-focused marketing and reach a wider audience with greater exposure over time are the ones that young people are most likely to use (Ross et al., 2015).

Eck said that the alcoholic beverage industry self-regulates its marketing, with the stated goal of protecting vulnerable populations, like youth. But, in reality, self-regulation is ineffective because brands do target youth and, for example, do advertise alcohol being used before or during risky activities, such as waterskiing and snowboarding (Noel et al., 2017). Eck highlighted an inherent tension between the industry's stated goal of protecting the youth and its business goal of building a future loyal customer base, which means marketing to the underage. One way of doing this, Eck said, is to produce a wide variety of alcoholic drinks that have been only available in nonalcoholic versions, such as lemonade, seltzer, soft drinks, and coffee.

Jessica Barrington-Trimis from the University of Southern California said that the tobacco industry also targets young people, describing how it uses different flavorings to do so. She said that most e-cigarettes are flavored, and flavors are a major reason that young people start vaping. Among young people who start vaping, 81–90 percent begin with a flavored product (Ambrose et al., 2015; Barrington-Trimis et al., 2024; Sargent et al., 2022). Barrington-Trimis and other speakers pointed out that the alcohol industry also uses flavored products to entice new users and create novel markets.

Pamela Ling from the University of California, San Francisco, discussed how tobacco companies extensively marketed their products in bars and nightclubs, where the industry has exploited reduced restrictions on marketing to people over the age of 21. Ling said that marketing to young adults who are using alcohol in these venues promotes tobacco use initiation, increased consumption, and co-use of both tobacco and alcohol (Ling and Glantz, 2002). The marketing included sponsoring bands and giving away merchandise, like free cigarettes, lip gloss, and branded accessories. Tobacco companies also use influencers on digital platforms to promote their products, said Ling, which expands the product's reach to young adults who do not frequent bars. Ling also pointed out that marketing tobacco products in bars reinforces the need to address the combined cancer-related health effects of using tobacco and alcohol together.[18]

Countering the Messaging from the Tobacco and Alcohol Industries

Adam Leventhal from the University of Southern California said that tobacco control policy interventions have, over the years, dramatically driven down the rate of cigarette use among 12th graders. From 1998 to 2024, their self-reported smoking prevalence decreased from 35 percent to 2.5 percent, or a decrease of 93 percent in the prevalence ratio (Miech et al., 2024). Leventhal noted that both tobacco and alcohol policies have tiered systems of regulatory oversight, from the federal government down to cities and other local municipalities. He added that for both substances, the greatest protections for youth occur at the local level. However, he said there are far more youth protections for tobacco products than for alcohol-containing beverages.

Leventhal identified four components of a youth-focused policy framework: regulating product characteristics, restricting marketing, limiting product access, and using warning labels. Leventhal provided several examples,

---

[18] The distribution of free samples of cigarettes was prohibited by the Family Smoking Prevention and Tobacco Control Act in 2009. However, there was an exception for e-cigarettes and some other smokeless products, which were prohibited after the 2016 Deeming Rule. See https://www.govinfo.gov/content/pkg/PLAW-111publ31/pdf/PLAW-111publ31.pdf and https://www.govinfo.gov/content/pkg/FR-2016-05-10/pdf/2016-10685.pdf (accessed July 29, 2025).

such as flavor additives in tobacco products, which are regulated to differing extents. The federal government allows only menthol as a cigarette flavor additive, but for 16 percent of the U.S. population, state and local governments ban menthol cigarettes. For e-cigarettes, menthol is the only flavor additive that the federal government allows,[19] while several state and local laws ban all flavored e-cigarette products, which covers about a quarter of the U.S. population. By contrast, there are no flavor additive restrictions on any alcoholic beverages, he said.

Leventhal noted that youth-focused control policies that have been implemented are effective at reducing substance use at a population level. These policies are generally more widely applied to tobacco than alcohol prevention. He urged researchers and regulators who specialize in either tobacco or alcohol to work collaboratively and learn from the successes and challenges that the other specialty has experienced.

In response to the overt presence of tobacco and alcohol promotion in bars and nightclubs, some artists, musicians, designers, and social marketers have pushed back with their own counter-marketing. Ling and colleagues evaluated the effectiveness of these efforts by performing time-location randomized sampling in bars before, during, and after a counter-marketing campaign. One effort in San Diego bars, over approximately 4 years, resulted in significant decreases in smoking prevalence and binge drinking among all target groups (Ling et al., 2014). In a similarly designed study in Oklahoma City, counter-marketing efforts over a 3-year period targeted people who frequented electronic dance music venues, Ling said. The survey results showed that young adults who recalled the smoke-free campaign had a notable decrease in smoking and a significant decrease in binge drinking (Fallin et al., 2015).

Several speakers emphasized that messaging about alcohol-related cancer risks cannot look the same as for tobacco-related cancer risks. Fong said that the messaging will differ because of the differences in how the two substances are perceived by the general public. Klein agreed and said that the relationships between socioeconomic status and the two substances are also quite different. He added that in the United States, alcohol is used across a broad spectrum of socioeconomic statuses, while tobacco use is more restricted to certain subpopulations. Fong suggested that to effectively counter marketing

---

[19] FDA released a policy on February 6, 2020, that enforces that flavored e-cigarettes, except menthol, cannot be sold in the United States. This was upheld in the Supreme Court on April 2, 2025. However, since this is an enforcement policy, flavored e-cigarettes may be available to purchase outside of these regulations. See https://www.fda.gov/regulatory-information/search-fda-guidance-documents/enforcement-priorities-electronic-nicotine-delivery-system-ends-and-other-deemed-products-market and https://www.supremecourt.gov/opinions/24pdf/23-1038_2d93.pdf (both accessed July 3, 2025).

and advertising efforts by the tobacco and alcohol industries, it is essential for health advocates and grassroots community organizations to use effective, trustworthy messaging and influence in structured ways.

Communicating the Impact of Tobacco and Alcohol Use on Cancer Risks and Related Health Outcomes to the Public

The public awareness of cancer-related health outcomes associated with tobacco use is higher in the United States compared to the awareness of outcomes associated with alcohol use. Hay said that one of the challenges to overcome when educating the public about these risks is the uncertainty of cancer risk; expressions of high uncertainty are related to low adherence with recommended health behaviors and high health information avoidance and associated with fatalism about cancer risk and a feeling of health information overload (Waters et al., 2022). For example, Hay said that messaging around the health risks of drinking alcohol is inconsistent. She explained that recent data indicate that when people self-report as being "moderate" drinkers, that can actually refer to consuming an amount of alcohol across a continuum from light to heavy drinking (Green et al., 2007; Gual et al., 2017; Pettigrew et al., 2017). This seems to be true in part because current public health messaging reinforces that moderate drinking is acceptable and does not increase one's cancer risk, Hay said. She suggested that public health information explaining the cancer-related risk of alcohol needs to promote informed decision making rather than focusing on abstinence and address the conflicting information about the putative beneficial effects of moderate alcohol consumption, appeal to shared values, give people positive goals, create community rather than division, and humanize the people who do the science and public health work behind these messages (Chou et al., 2025).

Several other speakers suggested some things to consider when developing a communication strategy about alcohol-related cancer risk. Berrigan said it is essential to use compelling infographics; focus on cancer risks of alcohol versus the other alcohol-related health risks; avoid comparisons with other modifiable risk factors, like smoking; educate people about and report both relative and absolute risk; and address the tension between the numerous risks of drinking alcohol. Amy Justice from Yale University and the Veterans Affairs Connecticut Healthcare System said that susceptibility to moderate levels of alcohol consumption varies by person and individual factors, such as age, family history, and health status. She added that it would be essential to be able to communicate to the public about multifactorial risk as well, because in reality, there are often multiple risk factors at play.

Eck said that translating the science into effective public health messaging can be a challenge. She added that the public wants the information about modifiable risk factors and their health effects, but it has to be provided in an understandable form so that people can see how it applies to them and members of their community and how they can be empowered to make changes that improve not only their own health but their community's health.

Shu-Hong Zhu from the University of California, San Diego, pointed out that an effective public health message around cigarettes has been that secondhand smoke harms the people around you. This message has helped drive smoke-free policies but also motivated smokers to change their behavior to avoid harming their children, for example. Zhu wondered whether an analogous set of messages could be developed for alcohol that would discourage underage drinking or target moderate and heavy drinkers by focusing on the impact on their loved ones.

Kolawole Okuyemi from the Indiana University School of Medicine pointed out that several years ago, some people working in tobacco research and policy decided to focus on elimination of all use of commercial tobacco products as the ultimate goal. He suggested that it would be beneficial for people in alcohol research and policy to also develop a clearly defined end goal. Okuyemi concurred when he said that for alcohol policies, it may not be to eliminate all drinking.

PREVENTION, CESSATION, AND REDUCTION EFFORTS

People who smoke, vape, drink alcohol, or use other tobacco products often have a time when they desire to quit. Benjamin Toll from the Medical University of South Carolina said that 68 percent of all people who vape plan to quit, and 64 percent of adults who both smoke and vape have wanted to quit (Palmer et al., 2021, 2024).[20,21] But quitting or switching to less harmful products is difficult and often requires multiple attempts. For example, less than 9 percent of adults who smoked and tried to quit in 2022 were successful, but nearly 67 percent of adults who have ever smoked cigarettes have quit for good.[22] Federal and state departments of health, along with private organizations like the ACS, provide resources like quitlines, other digital cessation tools, and access to cessation medications. Toll noted that many of the tools have been evaluated in randomized controlled trials and all use proven evidence-based methods to counsel and support people trying to quit or reduce harm.

---

[20] See CDC, Smoking and Tobacco Use, https://www.cdc.gov/tobacco/php/data-statistics/smoking-cessation/index.html (accessed May 29, 2025).

[21] Ibid.

[22] Ibid.

Quitlines and Other Digital Cessation Tools

Zhu said that California introduced the first statewide quitline in 1992, adding that it began as a telephone counseling service that could be accessed via a single telephone number from anywhere in the state. Its efficacy was evaluated in a randomized controlled trial, which showed that scheduled telephone sessions with a counselor using a structured protocol resulted in a greater number of people abstaining after their quit date than among the group who contacted the quitline but did not call back to request counseling (Zhu et al., 2002). By the end of 2004, all 50 states had established telephone-based counseling quitlines. Zhu said that creating quitlines across the United States and Canada led to the formation of the North American Quitline Consortium, whose mission is to help quitlines become more effective and more accessible.[23]

Zhu noted that quitlines have expanded in both the services delivered and types of counseling and support provided. For example, the New York quitline began mailing nicotine patches and gum to callers who requested them (Miller et al., 2005). He described a recent collaboration between the California quitline and the state's 211 service.[24] The goal was to reach a large swath of low-income people who use tobacco products and offer them cessation counseling. People referred to the quitline by 211 services were more than twice as likely to enroll in its services than were people referred by a health care professional or self-referred (Zhu et al., 2025).

Zhu said that by drawing on the current numerous digital resources that people access daily, quitlines could become "one-stop shops," providing counseling, support, information, and cessation medications. In addition to telehealth counseling, people have options to receive e-mails, texts, or online chatting; view videos and PDFs online; request medications; and receive AI-based counseling through their computers and cell phones. Zhu noted the need for continued monitoring and research to assess and test the efficacy of these various delivery modalities. He said that the success of tobacco quitlines provides some lessons on helping people who want to quit or reduce alcohol or cannabis use.

Toll discussed a 2015 randomized trial in which a quitline was used to counsel callers who both smoke and are heavy drinkers. Participants who received alcohol and tobacco counseling displayed a statistically significant higher rate of abstinence from smoking at their 7-month follow-up and reported fewer heavy drinking days in the week before the follow-up than

---

[23] See North American Quitline Consortium, https://www.naquitline.org/page/MissionGoalsVision (accessed April 30, 2025).

[24] See 211 California, https://211ca.org/ (accessed June 23, 2025).

did the group who received only tobacco counseling (Toll et al., 2015). Toll concluded that counseling can reduce alcohol consumption, adding that it is essential to leverage quitlines (among other tools) to counsel people who both smoke and drink heavily.

J. Lee Westmaas from ACS described the Empowered to Quit program,[25] which was created after a randomized controlled trial to assess the effectiveness of tailored e-mails for smoking cessation. The treatment group received 27 tailored e-mails over 6 weeks compared with a group that received three e-mails with links to cessation booklets and a group that received a single e-mail with a list of cessation resources. Participants in the treatment group had a significantly higher quit rate at their 6-month post-quit date than either of the two control groups (Westmaas et al., 2018). People sign up for the program on the ACS website and receive a welcome e-mail and a request to complete a short survey. Based on the information the user provides, it generates a series of tailored e-mails designed to support and prepare them for their quit attempt. E-mails arrive before and on the quit date and continue during the weeks afterward. Each message is tailored to provide support and resources to help them on their cessation journey.

Westmaas said that the Empowered to Quit program could be replicated to address alcohol use, noting that the first step is to determine if there is a demand for such a service. He said the components that can be replicated include identifying the triggers that cause people to drink; counseling on ways to mitigate, cope with, or avoid these; understanding the reasons why they want to change their drinking behavior; discussing available medication options; identifying cessation and behavior modification resources; and providing ongoing motivation, encouragement, and support.

Okuyemi identified six impediments to the effectiveness of smoking cessation programs and other tobacco control policy efforts. First, many people who smoke, especially from underserved communities, have difficulty accessing effective programs because of the cost, lack of insurance, and the absence of health care clinicians who specialize in tobacco use disorder. Second, Okuyemi said, lower levels of digital literacy among older adults and lower-income populations reduce their ability to use proven digital cessation tools. This problem is made worse by unequal distribution of broadband and cellular infrastructure nationwide. Third, for people who are trying to quit or have recently stopped smoking, the utility of e-cigarettes in harm reduction and smoking cessation efforts is affected by inconsistent regulations across many states. In addition, weak enforcement of smoke-free laws challenges people who are trying to quit. Fourth, relapse rates remain high, so it is essential

[25] See ACS Empowered to Quit, https://www.cancer.org/cancer/risk-prevention/tobacco/empowered-to-quit.html (accessed June 30, 2025).

to have better support measures and for longer periods after the quit date. Okuyemi said it would be helpful if smoking were thought of as a chronic disease that requires ongoing support and booster treatments. Fifth, people who consider quitting are exposed to misleading advertising by the tobacco industry, whose messages are designed to counter public health campaigns about the health risks. Sixth, tobacco control and cessation research and public health efforts continue to be underfunded compared with the public health costs. This impedes public health mass-reach efforts, the development of better cessation tools, and attempts to eliminate the health inequities surrounding tobacco use, Okuyemi said.

Pharmacological Cessation Approaches for Co-users

Babalola Faseru from the University of Kansas Medical Center said that the co-use of tobacco and alcohol is common and increases the morbidity and mortality risks from a variety of diseases, including cancer. Faseru added that it is important to treat them both to reduce the chance of substance relapse. He said that despite no FDA-approved medications to treat co-use, some medications have been shown in preliminary studies to be efficacious. Varenicline, a nicotinic acetylcholine partial receptor agonist, was shown to reduce both nicotine cravings and withdrawal symptoms while also decreasing alcohol consumption (Hurt et al., 2018). In a larger randomized controlled trial, varenicline combined with a nicotine patch given to people who smoke and also drank heavily resulted in significantly higher smoking abstinence levels than the control group who received only the patch (King et al., 2022). Both study groups showed significant decreases in drinking frequency. Unfortunately, the combination therapy also generated more adverse side effects; two participants (out of 61) required hospitalization, and five discontinued the treatment due to the adverse effects (King et al., 2022). Faseru said that glucagon-like peptide-1 (GLP-1) receptor agonists, which are FDA-approved for Type 2 diabetes and weight management, affect pathways in the brain's reward system that are also influenced by nicotine and alcohol. In one small randomized controlled trial, participants who received a GLP-1 receptor agonist (semaglutide) showed a 41 percent decrease in alcohol intake compared with the control group and also a steady decline in cigarettes smoked per day over 9 weeks (Hendershot et al., 2025). A larger randomized controlled trial assessed the effectiveness of combining nicotine replacement therapy with another GLP-1 receptor agonist (exenatide) to avoid significant weight gain. Participants who were given exenatide along with nicotine patches and counseling showed reduced cravings and withdrawal symptoms, improved smoking abstinence, and reduced weight gain among those who were able to abstain from smoking compared with the control group (Yammine et al., 2021).

Tailoring Interventions to Underserved Communities

Ella Greene-Moton from the American Public Health Association (APHA) said that the effectiveness of tobacco prevention and cessation strategies depends on the involvement of the community. Therefore, to do community-based participatory research, grassroots community members need to first feel that they are welcome at the table; that they can understand and trust the messages and the evidence that are being presented by researchers and clinicians; and, importantly, that the language used by the researchers is culturally appropriate and not offensive to them. She added that "it's about creating spaces to create relationships [and] to create partnerships."

Greene-Moton said that tobacco and alcohol use contribute significantly to cancer-related health disparities and a higher incidence of chronic diseases. She noted that APHA, for example, partners with federal, state, and local organizations to address such disparities by working with policy makers to develop smoke-free laws and policies, increase taxes on tobacco, and develop and disseminate public education campaigns concerning the health risks of smoking. She added that APHA supports a similar agenda for alcohol-related prevention and developing educational materials to raise awareness about alcohol-related cancer risk, advocating for higher taxes on alcoholic beverages, and advocating for restrictions on alcohol advertising. "APHA's efforts seek to remedy the health disparities and disadvantages that marginalized communities confront every day," Greene-Moton concluded.

Francisco Cartujano-Barrera from the University of Rochester Medical Center also highlighted the differences in outcomes across different populations and emphasized the importance of involving the community in research. He explained that members of the community can serve on advisory boards to provide input and guidance on identifying health concerns, collaborate in shared decision making, engage in intervention design, guide recruitment strategies, participate in recruitment efforts, and assist in interpreting and disseminating the results.

Cartujano-Barrera said that smoking prevalence among Latinos broadly is 8 percent, one of the lowest rates for a racial or ethnic group (Cornelius, 2022). However, subdividing Latinos by national background revealed significant heterogeneity. Among Cubans and Puerto Ricans, it is as high as 40 percent, depending on the age cohort (Kaplan et al., 2014). Furthermore, Latinos disproportionately experience poor health and health outcomes, with reduced access to cessation counseling and medications and fewer opportunities to participate in cessation studies (Cartujano-Barrera et al., 2019; de Dios et al., 2019; VanFrank et al., 2024).

Cartujano-Barrera described a culturally and linguistically appropriate text messaging tool, *Decídetexto*, that was designed by and for U.S. Latino communities to aid in smoking cessation. He said that in a randomized controlled study to assess its efficacy, participants were significantly more likely to be abstinent at months 3 and 6 than people in the control group were (Cartujano-Barrera et al., 2020, 2025). Due to the success of this and several other community-based participatory research efforts in Latino communities, Cartujano-Barrera explained that he and his colleagues developed a culturally and linguistically appropriate toolkit for the American Lung Association to help strengthen the knowledge of health care professionals, public health workers, educators, public officials, community and faith-based organizations, and others regarding tobacco use, prevention, and cessation to better serve Hispanic or Latino communities.[26]

Ayana Jordan from the New York University Grossman School of Medicine emphasized that effective community-based participatory research is done with communities rather than in or on them. Jordan said that the Imani Breakthrough project, which she began with colleagues in New Haven, Connecticut, incorporated a faith-based recovery initiative targeting Black and Latino community members with opioid use disorder.[27] The program began with 12 weeks of classes and activities focused on wellness enhancement and helping participants to become engaged in the community. These efforts were supported by trained staff who assisted participants in reaching their recovery and reintegration goals. The initial 12 weeks were followed by a 10-week mutual support program to further assist participants in goal setting, reaching goals, and addressing challenges like food or housing insecurity. Jordan said that each of the 808 participants saw improvements by every measure of wellness, community engagement, and traditional substance use disorder outcomes (Bellamy et al., 2021).

Jordan described another study focused on Black adults with AUD, using evidence-based treatments provided in Black churches rather than traditional clinics. Recruitment within the community was facilitated by a pastor. The study provided evidence that an 8-week alcohol treatment in a nontraditional setting could provide positive results, as measured by follow-ups at 3, 6, and 12 months (Jordan et al., 2021). Notably, Jordan added, the treatment methodology included a focus on spirituality and prayer, along with time for relaxation and reflection, which helped build support and motivation in the recovery process.

---

[26] See Addressing Tobacco Use in Hispanic or Latino Communities Toolkit, American Lung Association, https://www.lung.org/getmedia/1063c716-425d-4684-8647-14a37a72580a/Hispanic_Latino_Communities_Toolkit_ENG.pdf (accessed May 19, 2025).

[27] See Imani Breakthrough project, https://portal.ct.gov/dmhas/newsworthy/news-items/the-imani-breakthrough-project (accessed June 23, 2025).

Melissa Buffalo from the American Indian Cancer Foundation said that cancer is the second leading cause of death among American Indian and Alaska Native (AIAN) people, behind cardiovascular disease (CDC, 2025). Buffalo added that Alaska Native people have the highest incidence of and mortality rate for colorectal cancer in the world, and among various U.S. demographic groups, the AIAN population has the highest incidence of cervical, colorectal, kidney, liver, and lung cancers (Nash et al., 2021; White et al., 2014).

Indigenous peoples recognize two types of tobacco: commercial and traditional. The former causes sickness, disease, and death. Buffalo said that "traditional medicine is healing for us and is something that is part of our life every day." She pointed out that traditional tobacco is not smoked; it is instead prepared and used as medicine, offerings, and gifts. It is integral to American Indian culture, alongside Native languages, religions, and values. Buffalo stressed that commercial tobacco, however, is killing Indigenous people. She said that SmokefreeNATIVE,[28] a culturally focused cessation program, was created to address the health risks and addiction of commercial tobacco while honoring the importance and significance of traditional tobacco.

Buffalo said that among Indigenous populations, the use of alcohol and commercial tobacco, along with limited access to health care and high rates of poverty, "are the result of official U.S. colonization, forced displacement, violence, and suppression of Native culture across more than 200 years" (John-Henderson et al., 2023).

Buffalo said that the American Indian Cancer Foundation educates Indigenous people about other cancers as well, like breast and liver cancers. The foundation outreach explains what modifiable risk factors are and how to successfully quit using commercial tobacco, reduce alcohol consumption, moderate weight, expand exercise, and address stress.

Cessation Treatment Following a Cancer Diagnosis

Graham Warren from the Medical University of South Carolina[29] said that while it is widely known that smoking tobacco is strongly associated with the risk of developing cancer, for people who have received a cancer diagnosis, that message too often trails off. But, Warren said, "if you continue to smoke after a cancer diagnosis, the effects of smoking don't go away." A 2014 surgeon general's report on the health consequences concluded that patients with can-

[28] SmokefreeNATIVE was developed by experts at the University of Minnesota School of Public Health and the American Indian Cancer Foundation in collaboration with the Indian Health Service and the National Cancer Institute's (NCI's) Smokefree.gov initiative.

[29] Dr. Warren is currently at the University of Kentucky College of Medicine.

cer and cancer survivors who continued to smoke increased their risks of overall and cancer-related mortality by 50 and 60 percent, respectively, compared with people who never smoked and nonsmokers (HHS, 2014). The report also concluded that smoking cigarettes was "consistently strongly associated with poorer responses to treatment, with evidence of a dose-response trend of worse response with more extensive smoking" (HHS, 2014, p. 290). Warren stressed that integrating smoking cessation into cancer treatment creates an opportunity to affect the "biologic, clinical, and value-based outcomes" (Warren and Simmons, 2023; Warren et al., 2014b). Smoking after a cancer diagnosis also has large economic effects, he said. Warren and colleagues estimated that the cost of cancer treatment in the United States attributable to continued smoking after diagnosis was approximately $3.4 billion annually (2019 estimates). They focused solely on the expenses related to the administration of second-, third-, and fourth-line drugs that become necessary because smoking increases the risk of first-line treatment failure (Warren et al., 2019).

Warren said that the survival improvements after smoking cessation are comparable to those that followed the introduction of contemporary cancer treatment including immunotherapies. He noted the need for innovation in the tobacco cessation methods and that many agents and approaches in use are 30 years old. He advocated for developing more effective pharmacologic agents and increasing access to cessation tools, medications, and counseling. Warren also pointed out that engaging patients early in the diagnostic process and using "positive messaging" are valuable ways to help patients and their families understand the value of quitting tobacco and empower them to work together toward achievable health outcomes.

Warren and colleagues instituted one of the first opt-out smoking cessation programs specifically for patients with cancer (Warren et al., 2014a). About 12,000 patients were screened using a structured assessment, and active smokers were automatically referred to a telephone-based program. Patients who quit smoking while participating had a 44 percent reduction in lung cancer mortality compared with patients who did not (Dobson Amato et al., 2015). A few years later, the researchers evaluated whether the timing of entry into a tobacco cessation program following a cancer diagnosis impacted the survival rate. They found that survival outcomes were optimal for patients who achieved cessation within 6 months of diagnosis resulting in an approximate 4-year improvement in median survival as compared with patients who continued to smoke, emphasizing the importance of early postdiagnosis entry into an evidence-based program (Cinciripini et al., 2024).

Based on the evidence that smoking cessation improves cancer outcomes and increases the life-span after a lung cancer diagnosis, the National Comprehensive Cancer Network and NCI, in collaboration with the American

Association for Cancer Research, have funded additional related research and also developed guidelines designed to improve the process of helping people with a cancer diagnosis to quit smoking and facilitate assessment of smoking in the context of cancer research and treatment.[30] Three U.S. and Canadian initiatives have also integrated smoking cessation into clinical cancer centers, involving thousands of central and community cancer centers and enrolling hundreds of thousands of patients.[31] Warren said that accrediting policy and guideline organizations have a key role in incorporating smoking cessation into cancer care and concluded, "We have the opportunity to address smoking across the continuum of cancer care, and that will give us the opportunity to have a consistent message to all patients and in all cancer treatment settings that quitting smoking even after a cancer diagnosis can make a big difference."

Approaches to Vaping Cessation

Toll reported that in 2025, smoke-free nicotine products will surpass, by volume, the consumption of combustible tobacco products (Herzog et al., 2025). This is consistent with data showing that from 2013 through 2021, among young adults aged 18–24, the prevalence of smoking declined but that of vaping increased (Sanford et al., 2024). Toll said that despite the rise in e-cigarette use, more than 77 percent of people who vape exclusively also plan to quit (Palmer et al., 2021, 2024). He added that these results point to a need to expand research, cessation assistance, and nicotine control policies that focus on e-cigarettes and other noncombustible tobacco products. Freedman agreed and said that it is very important to further research into e-cigarettes as their use increases.

Toll said that in one pilot study, e-cigarette users were randomized to three groups, each receiving nicotine replacement therapy, varying in the amount of nicotine provided (Palmer et al., 2025). The mid- and high-dose groups showed the same rates of abstinence at days 28 and 56, but the mid-dose therapy had fewer side effects. In another randomized controlled study, the group of e-cigarette users who were given varenicline had a significantly higher quit rate at weeks 8 and 12 compared to the placebo control group

---

[30] See National Comprehensive Cancer Network Guidelines, https://www.nccn.org/guidelines/guidelines-detail (accessed July 3, 2025).

[31] See Cancer Center Cessation Initiative, https://cancercontrol.cancer.gov/brp/tcrb/cancer-center-cessation-initiative; Canadian Partnership Against Cancer, https://www.partnershipagainstcancer.ca/; and American College of Surgeons Commission on Cancer Just ASK and Beyond ASK programs, https://www.facs.org/quality-programs/cancer-programs/cancer-qi-programs/pdsa-just-ask/ and https://www.facs.org/quality-programs/cancer-programs/cancer-qi-programs/beyond-ask-quality-improvement-project/ (all sites accessed May 29, 2025).

(Fucito et al., 2024). Toll said that while these results are promising, more studies are needed to develop efficacious cessation tools for assisting e-cigarette users and people who both smoke and vape.

When asked about the harms caused by vaping compared with smoking-induced health problems, Faseru responded that vaping exposes users to fewer toxicants than smoking. He added that studies have shown that for people who have been unable to quit, vaping is helpful as a harm reduction tool and can help people to reduce or even quit smoking. Both Faseru and Toll said that switching from smoking to vaping may be challenging due to potential for dual use and its associated risks. Ling noted that despite the reduced exposure to toxins when vaping compared with smoking, many observational cohort studies link vaping to pulmonary and cardiovascular disease, but much fewer data link it to cancer. She added that epigenomic studies of DNA damage associated with cancer risk show little difference between the changes that result from smoking or from e-cigarette use (Tommasi et al., 2023, 2025).

Tobacco Prevention for the Youth Population

Ling agreed with King that the vast majority of tobacco smoking initiation occurs in the youth population. She added that among high school students, the most prevalent substances used are alcohol, e-cigarettes, and cannabis. Ling explained that young people start for personal reasons but are also influenced by peers, social norms, industry marketing, and structural elements like control policies, social determinants of health, and discrimination. Ling said that following the release of the 1964 surgeon general's report on the health effects of smoking, more than 130 school-based antitobacco programs were implemented to encourage youth not to smoke or to quit, including 50 randomized controlled trials (Thomas et al., 2015). Studies showed evidence of effectiveness, particularly for programs that were able to provide follow-up with youth for over 1 year (Thomas et al., 2015). When all trials or trials with follow-up beyond 1 year were pooled, the programs reduced smoking initiation by 12 percent (Thomas et al., 2015).

In addition, Ling noted that some school-based alcohol prevention programs have shown evidence of effectiveness (Spoth et al., 2008). She said that despite many intervention programs designed for college students, most aim to moderate alcohol use rather than encouraging prevention and cessation, with far fewer focused on tobacco use. She noted the opportunity to conduct more research on tobacco and alcohol program crossover effects.

CHALLENGES AND OPPORTUNITIES TO REDUCE TOBACCO- AND ALCOHOL-RELATED CANCER RISK

Addressing Stigma and Perception Bias

Gwen Darien from the Patient Advocate Foundation said that people with a cancer diagnosis frequently deal with stigma, blame, and uncertainty. She said that after her first diagnosis, people would ask her what she thought she had done to get cancer. She noted that this both ascribes blame to the person with the diagnosis and implies that it was somehow avoidable. Darien said that at the core of stigma, blame, and uncertainty lies the issue of trust. If people do not trust their health care professional or the health care system, then they are less likely to get screened or see a clinician regularly. This is especially true with stigmatized conditions, she added.

Lisa Carter-Bawa from the Cancer Prevention Precision Control Institute agreed with Darien and stressed the great deal of stigma and blame around smoking. Carter-Bawa said, "Until we address stigma, we are never going to effectively support patients, promote early detection, or achieve any semblance of significant advancements in treatment outcomes." She noted that lung cancer stigma can negatively impact cancer treatment outcomes by reducing the sense of self-worth, exacerbating depression and anxiety, and reducing treatment adherence (Carter-Bawa et al., 2023). Lung cancer stigma has been reported by 95 percent of people with the diagnosis, including nearly half of those people hearing it from their health care clinicians (Hamann et al., 2014; Shen et al., 2016). Carter-Bawa said that as long as people who smoke are blamed with no recognition that smoking is an addiction, stigmatization will persist, and all of its negative consequences will flourish.

Carter-Bawa suggested that to overcome stigmatization, it would be helpful to change the public discourse, stop using messaging that demonizes people who smoke, and shift to empathic methods. She noted that empathic communication is associated with higher levels of patient treatment compliance and lower levels of psychological distress and that good patient–clinician communication is associated with lower levels of stigma. Carter-Bawa concluded that public health messaging should be hope-filled and inspiring or simply nonjudgmental.

Gail Eckhardt from Baylor College of Medicine asked how clinicians, especially oncologists, can talk with their patients about the cancer risks from drinking alcohol in a way that is free of guilt and blame. Darien suggested talking about risk in the same manner that health care professionals use for treatment decisions: by focusing on shared decision making. She added that when the conversation is centered on shared decision making and shared behavior, with no implicit or explicit blame, then the patient is not stigmatized and the patient–health care professional bond strengthens. Justice added that communicating risk, which is a complicated problem, is necessary but may not be sufficient if a patient is not motivated to alter behavior. She said that it is important to personalize the conversation for each individual patient.

Carter-Bawa said that to avoid stigmatizing people who use alcohol, it is essential for public health messaging to use person-centered language that does not treat behavior as the problem but rather acknowledges the addictive nature of substances and portrays alcohol use as a risk factor for certain cancers and other health problems. Leventhal agreed and said that public health messaging and the patient–clinician conversations can make the substance less glamorous without attaching a stigma to the person. Okuyemi pointed out that the messaging may need to differ depending on the target audience. He said that the fear and shock approach was effective decades ago, but motivational and positive approaches are the more effective strategies today.

Toll said that some patients do not want to be screened for lung cancer for fear that they gave themselves cancer. He asked about any interventions to mitigate this self-directed stigma. Carter-Bawa responded that her group has created a computer-based communication and decision support tool to educate users about the value of lung cancer screening and encourage them to get screened if a clinician recommends it.[32] It is also used after screening to provide cessation support to the patient, acknowledging that breaking a habit is a journey that requires time and sustained support.

Robert Winn from the Virginia Commonwealth University agreed that technology in the clinic and in clinical research can be enormously useful but cautioned that it is important to also cultivate the human connection. He said that a rise in isolation and loneliness and a reduction in social gatherings is making it harder for people to find sources of trusted information. Winn urged clinicians and researchers to find ways to expand community outreach and engagement and meet people within their communities.

Lessons Learned from Studies Within the U.S. Veterans Health Care System

Justice said that to properly understand the impacts of alcohol and tobacco use on cancer risk and outcomes, researchers need adequate sample sizes and should move beyond self-reported measures of exposure and account for the time delay between exposure and cancer and the reality that many people use multiple substances, which impacts the analysis.

---

[32] For more information, please see LungTalk: https://www.lungtalkhmh.org/ (accessed May 29, 2025).

Justice noted that the U.S. Veterans Health Administration is an extraordinary resource for researchers because it is the largest U.S. integrated health care system, represents more than 13 million people, possesses electronic health records dating back to 1998, maintains a cancer registry, and has extensive data on smoking and alcohol use, pharmacy use, and mortality (Golden et al., 2020; Na et al., 2023; Zullig et al., 2024). Because self-reporting of alcohol and tobacco use may be prone to underreporting, social desirability bias, and abstainer bias, Justice recommended measuring DNA methylation as an unbiased biomarker of tobacco use, which also has the advantage of reflecting longer-term exposure. The gold standard biomarker for alcohol use is phosphatidyl ethanol because it unmasks any social desirability bias, she said. Justice said that biomarker tests are also preferable because of a racial bias with the Alcohol Use Disorders Identification Test—Consumption. One study of more than 700,000 veterans found that Black and Hispanic veterans were given an AUD diagnosis at higher rates than White veterans, despite having similar levels of consumption based on the test (Vickers-Smith et al., 2023).

Many people among the general public are unaware that there is a multiyear delay between quitting either tobacco or alcohol and the return to a baseline value of cancer risk. For example, it takes more than 10 years after quitting smoking to eliminate tobacco as a risk factor for lung cancer,[33] and it may take 20 years after a person stops drinking alcohol before the risk of alcohol-based hepatocellular cancer disappears (Heckley et al., 2011).

Gaps in Economic Research and Taxation Policy

Based on a review of evidence of the effectiveness of U.S. alcohol taxation policy, Nigar Nargis from ACS reported that there is ample evidence to suggest that tax-induced price increases can reduce alcohol consumption and associated health risks. Nargis said an increase in the excise tax would be the most cost-effective method, as measured by dollars spent per healthy life years gained. Nargis suggested that the tax rate should be proportional to the societal costs of drinking, such as negative impacts to public health, domestic violence, motor vehicle accidents, and violent crime. Nargis noted a need for more research to quantitate appropriate tax rates based on the health costs of consumption, but based on various models, she said the 2024-adjusted tax should be around $1.34–1.40 per ounce of pure alcohol (Herrnstadt et al., 2015; Manning et al., 1989). This greatly exceeds the current average combined tax rate of $0.25 per ounce.

[33] See ACS Health Benefits of Quitting Smoking Over Time, https://www.cancer.org/cancer/risk-prevention/tobacco/guide-quitting-smoking/benefits-of-quitting-smoking-over-time.html (accessed May 24, 2025).

Nargis and Drope said that increasing taxes and concomitant increases in the price of alcohol reduce demand, but a recent systematic review of studies that looked at the effect of price increases on consumption identified a number of evidence gaps (Guindon et al., 2022). The key findings of the review showed that most studies are relatively out-of-date because the array of beverages is quite different from what was available when these studies were published and the studies do not differentiate among low, moderate, and heavy drinking; consider the impacts of switching products in response to price increases; or examine the evidence for reducing consumption (e.g., heavy to moderate drinking) due to price increases. Nargis said that it would also be useful to have more studies that tease out the effect of alcohol taxes on consumption based on demographic factors, like income, race, ethnicity, gender identity, education, and occupational status (Kilian et al., 2023). Nargis concluded by reiterating that this economic research should not be siloed; rather, alcohol tax policy should be examined within the nexus of unhealthy products (alcohol, tobacco, cannabis, sweetened drinks, illegal and prescription drugs, and ultraprocessed foods) because people may consume or use multiple products from this set, and as pricing policies change, people may switch from one unhealthy product to another.

Drope, Nargis, and Ribisl said that excise taxes are most effective at reducing consumption when they are combined with other tools, like a minimum price and bans on promotions and discounts at the point of sale. Drope said research has shown that young people reduce consumption of tobacco products when prices increase, but the evidence is mixed about their response for alcoholic beverages (Guindon et al., 2022). This is an area where more research would be helpful, he said. Drope noted the structural differences between the taxation of tobacco and alcohol and behavioral differences in consumer responses to price changes in these two types of goods, so more research is needed to effectively craft policy that uses alcohol taxation as a fiscal and public health tool.

Faseru asked whether states could assemble a legal challenge against the alcohol industry similar to the ones that resulted in the Master Settlement Agreement against the tobacco industry. Leventhal responded that attorneys general would have to decide to pursue that litigation and have a compelling legal argument. Leventhal noted that the attorneys general argued that the tobacco industry had misled the public for years about the health effects of cigarettes, and if a similar situation existed for the alcohol industry, that could be a place to begin. Leventhal also said that effective mass-reach public health messaging about alcohol-related cancer risks is essential for shifting the public's attitude and behavior, which propels changes in policy and litigation. Toll said that litigation is a public health strategy and identified several reasons why it is a useful avenue to pursue with alcohol: it can lead to significant penalties levied against the industry, which can be used to further alcohol control efforts; it forces document disclosure by the industry, exposing its misdeeds and transforming public health campaigns; and all of these efforts and transformations propel policy changes that strengthen alcohol policy efforts.

Expanding Research on Co-use of Substances

Justice said that people who smoke are more likely than nonsmokers to use a second substance, such as alcohol, opioids, cannabis, cocaine, or amphetamines (Moeller et al., 2018; Richter et al., 2017), so "we really need to get beyond thinking about just alcohol and tobacco—we need to think about the whole picture of what people are doing, especially with this aging population where marijuana use is very common." She added that among people over 60, many are taking multiple prescribed medications and using other psychoactive substances, including alcohol, tobacco, cannabis, and cocaine (HHS, 2020b).

A recent systematic review found limited evidence on the association of cannabis as a risk factor for cancer (Nargis et al., 2025), and now that cannabis use is legal or decriminalized in the vast majority of states, research on its cancer risk is needed, said Barrington-Trimis. She emphasized the value and importance of understanding how tobacco, alcohol, and cannabis use—especially among young people—overlap and how co-use impacts health risks. Barrington-Trimis gave examples of marketing that blurs the line between tobacco products, like e-cigarettes and smokeless tobacco, and cannabis products. She said that these similarities encourage young people to move between the use of these different, but similar looking, products. Similarly, she said that beverages infused with tetrahydrocannabinol are marketed as replacements for other beverages, both alcoholic and nonalcoholic. Barrington-Trimis said that there is also a need for research on the co-use of alcohol, tobacco, and cannabis to inform policy makers that can lead to more comprehensive and effective policy. She highlighted the need for evidence-based policy that considers the impacts of these three products on users across the life-span. Berrigan said that research comparing alcohol and cannabis could be useful because both substances are reported to have a mix of positive and negative health effects. Jordan said that smoking tobacco and cannabis together leads to significant adverse health effects (Hindocha and McClure, 2021).

CLOSING THOUGHTS

The session co-moderators summarized the key messages to spur progress toward a deeper understanding of the effects of both tobacco and alcohol and suggested actions from participants to mitigate the risks of alcohol and tobacco use that emerged from their sessions (see Boxes 1 and 2). Winn urged clinicians, researchers, and policy makers that it is essential to engage users of tobacco and alcohol through community-informed, culturally sensitive messaging that avoids stigma and fosters trust by combining human connection with thoughtful use of technology.

References

AICR (American Institute for Cancer Research). 2019. *2019 AICR Cancer Risk Awareness Survey.* Washington, DC: American Institute for Cancer Research. https://www.aicr.org/assets/can-prevent/docs/2019-Survey.pdf (accessed July 30, 2025).

Ambrose, B. K., H. R. Day, B. Rostron, K. P. Conway, N. Borek, A. Hyland, and A. C. Villanti. 2015. Flavored tobacco product use among U.S. youth aged 12–17 years, 2013–2014. *JAMA* 314(17):1871–1873.

Barrington-Trimis, J. L., M. Stoolmiller, E. A. Vogel, A. Harlow, A. P. Tackett, J. B. Unger, R. McConnell, A. M. Leventhal, J. Audrain-McGovern, and J. D. Sargent. 2024. Recall of flavor at first e-cigarette use and its association with e-cigarette progression: The mediating effects of first sensory experience. *Journal of Pediatrics* 275:114246.

Bellamy, C. D., M. Costa, J. Wyatt, M. Mathis, A. Sloan, M. Budge, K. Blackman, L. Ocasio, G. Reis, K. Guy, Rev. R. Anderson, M. Stewart Copes, and A. Jordan. 2021. A collaborative culturally-centered and community-driven faith-based opioid recovery initiative: The Imani Breakthrough project. *Social Work in Mental Health* 19(6):558–567.

Blanchette, J. G., M. C. Lira, T. C. Heeren, and T. S. Naimi. 2020. Alcohol policies in U.S. states, 1999–2018. *Journal of Studies on Alcohol and Drugs* 81(1):58–67.

Brewer, N. T., M. G. Hall, S. M. Noar, H. Parada, A. Stein-Seroussi, L. E. Bach, S. Hanley, and K. M. Ribisl. 2016. Effect of pictorial cigarette pack warnings on changes in smoking behavior: A randomized clinical trial. *JAMA Internal Medicine* 176(7):905–912.

Burris, J. L., T. N. Borger, B. J. Shelton, A. K. Darville, J. L. Studts, J. Valentino, C. Blair, D. B. Davis, and J. Scales. 2022. Tobacco use and tobacco treatment referral response of patients with cancer: Implementation outcomes at a National Cancer Institute-designated cancer center. *JCO Oncology Practice* 18(2):e261–e270.

Califf, R. M., and B. A. King. 2023. The need for a smoking cessation "care package." *JAMA* 329(3):203–204.

Carter-Bawa, L., J. S. Ostroff, K. Hoover, and J. L. Studts. 2023. Effective communication about lung cancer screening without iatrogenic stigma: A brief report case study using the Lung Cancer Stigma Communications Assessment Tool of LungTalk. *JTO Clinical and Research Reports* 4(11):100585.

Cartujano-Barrera, F., J. Perales, E. Arana, L. S. Cox, H. W. Yeh, E. F. Ellerbeck, K. P. Richter, and A. P. Cupertino. 2019. Increasing access to smoking cessation treatment among Latino smokers using case management. *Journal of Smoking Cessation* 14(3):168–175.

Cartujano-Barrera, F., E. Arana-Chicas, D. Catley, L. Sanderson Cox, F. J. Diaz, E. F. Ellerbeck, K. D. Graves, C. Ogedegbe, and A. P. Cupertino. 2020. Decídetexto: Mobile cessation support for Latino smokers: Study protocol for a randomized clinical trial. *Contemporary Clinical Trials* 99:106188.

Cartujano-Barrera, F., L. S. Cox, D. Catley, X. Cai, F. J. Diaz, E. Arana-Chicas, A. Chávez-Iñiguez, C. Ogedegbe, K. D. Graves, M. P. Rivera, A. Ponce, E. F. Ellerbeck, and A. P. Cupertino. 2025. Decídetexto: Mobile cessation support for Latino adults who smoke: A randomized clinical trial. *Chest* 167(2):619–629.

CDC (Centers for Disease Control and Prevention). 2024. *Current Cigarette Smoking Among Adults in the United States*. https://www.cdc.gov/tobacco/php/data-statistics/adult-data-cigarettes/index.html (accessed June 20, 2025).

CDC. 2025. *State Tobacco Activities Tracking and Evaluation (STATE) System*. https://www.cdc.gov/statesystem/index.html (accessed June 20, 2025).

Chaffee, B. W., C. D. Donaldson, E. T. Couch, C. Guerra Castillo, O. Farooq, N. F. Cheng, N. Ameli, M. L. Wilkinson, S. A. Gansky, X. Zhang, and K. S. Hoeft. 2025. Flavored tobacco product use among California adolescents before and immediately after a statewide flavor ban. *Nicotine & Tobacco Research* 27(6):1035–1042.

Chakraborty, R., M. L. Berman, Y. T. Yang, Y. Li, Y. Wang, D. Bernat, S. Zhang, and C. J. Berg. 2025. State preemption and local tobacco control: Constraints and opportunities for innovation in the U.S. *International Journal of Environmental Research and Public Health* 22(6):827.

Chou, W. S., I. A. Iles, A. Gaysynsky, and W. M. P. Klein. 2025. Public health communication approaches for building common ground. *American Journal of Public Health* 115(4):511–518.

Cinciripini, P. M., G. Kypriotakis, J. A. Blalock, M. Karam-Hage, D. M. Beneventi, J. D. Robinson, J. A. Minnix, and G. W. Warren. 2024. Survival outcomes of an early intervention smoking cessation treatment after a cancer diagnosis. *JAMA Oncology* 10(12):1689–1696.

Cornelius, M. E. 2022. Tobacco product use among adults—United States, 2020. *MMWR* 71(11):397–405.

de Dios, M. A., M. Á. Cano, E. L. Vaughan, S. D. Childress, M. M. McNeel, L. M. Harvey, and R. S. Niaura. 2019. A pilot randomized trial examining the feasibility and acceptability of a culturally tailored and adherence-enhancing intervention for Latino smokers in the U.S. *PLOS ONE* 14(1):e0210323.

Dobson Amato, K. A., A. Hyland, R. Reed, M. C. Mahoney, J. Marshall, G. Giovino, M. Bansal-Travers, H. M. Ochs-Balcom, M. A. Zevon, K. M. Cummings, C. Nwogu, A. K. Singh, H. Chen, G. W. Warren, and M. Reid. 2015. Tobacco cessation may improve lung cancer patient survival. *Journal of Thoracic Oncology* 10(7):1014–1019.

Fallin, A., T. B. Neilands, J. W. Jordan, J. S. Hong, and P. M. Ling. 2015. Wreaking "havoc" on smoking: Social branding to reach young adult "partiers" in Oklahoma. *American Journal of Preventive Medicine* 48(1 Suppl 1):S78–85.

Fong, G. T., D. Hammond, and S. C. Hitchman. 2009. The impact of pictures on the effectiveness of tobacco warnings. *Bulletin World Health Organization* 87(8):640–643.

Fucito, L. M., S. R. Baldassarri, N. L. Baker, A. M. Palmer, S. S. O'Malley, M. J. Carpenter, S. Krishnan-Sarin, K. M. Gray, and B. A. Toll. 2024. Varenicline for e-cigarette cessation in adults: A preliminary placebo-controlled randomized trial. *American Journal of Preventive Medicine* 67(2):296–298.

Gapstur, S. M., V. Bouvard, S. T. Nethan, J. L. Freudenheim, C. C. Abnet, D. R. English, J. Rehm, S. Balbo, P. Buykx, and D. Crabb. 2023. The IARC perspective on alcohol reduction or cessation and cancer risk. *New England Journal of Medicine* 389(26):2486–2494.

Golden, S. D., M. C. Farrelly, D. A. Luke, and K. M. Ribisl. 2016. Comparing projected impacts of cigarette floor price and excise tax policies on socioeconomic disparities in smoking. *Tobacco Control* 25(Suppl 1):i60–i66.

Golden, S. E., E. R. Hooker, S. Shull, M. Howard, K. Crothers, R. F. Thompson, and C. G. Slatore. 2020. Validity of Veterans Health Administration structured data to determine accurate smoking status. *Health Informatics Journal* 26(3):1507–1515.

Green, A. C., P. Driezen, S. M. Noar, D. Hammond, and G. T. Fong. 2019. Impact of adding and removing warning label messages from cigarette packages on adult smokers' awareness about the health harms of smoking: Findings from the ITC Canada survey. *Tobacco Control* 28(e1):e56–e63.

Green, C. A., M. R. Polen, S. L. Janoff, D. K. Castleton, and N. A. Perrin. 2007. "Not getting tanked": Definitions of moderate drinking and their health implications. *Drug and Alcohol Dependence* 86(2-3):265–273.

Gual, A., J. Ángel Arbesú, J. Zarco, M. L. M. Balcells-Oliveró, H. López-Pelayo, L. Miquel, and J. Bobes. 2017. Risky drinkers underestimate their own alcohol consumption. *Alcohol and Alcoholism* 52(4):516–517.

Guindon, G. E., K. Zhao, T. Fatima, S. Garasia, N. Quinn, N. B. Baskerville, and G. Paraje. 2022. Prices, taxes and alcohol use: A systematic umbrella review. *Addiction* 117(12):3004–3023.

Hamann, H. A., J. S. Ostroff, E. G. Marks, D. E. Gerber, J. H. Schiller, and S. J. Lee. 2014. Stigma among patients with lung cancer: A patient-reported measurement model. *Psychooncology* 23(1):81–92.

Hashibe, M., P. Brennan, S. C. Chuang, S. Boccia, X. Castellsague, C. Chen, M. P. Curado, L. Dal Maso, A. W. Daudt, E. Fabianova, L. Fernandez, V. Wünsch-Filho, S. Franceschi, R. B. Hayes, R. Herrero, K. Kelsey, S. Koifman, C. La Vecchia, P. Lazarus, F. Levi, J. J. Lence, D. Mates, E. Matos, A. Menezes, M. D. McClean, J. Muscat, J. Eluf-Neto, A. F. Olshan, M. Purdue, P. Rudnai, S. M. Schwartz, E. Smith, E. M. Sturgis, N. Szeszenia-Dabrowska, R. Talamini, Q. Wei, D. M. Winn, O. Shangina, A. Pilarska, Z. F. Zhang, G. Ferro, J. Berthiller, and P. Boffetta. 2009. Interaction between tobacco and alcohol use and the risk of head and neck cancer: Pooled analysis in the International Head and Neck Cancer Epidemiology Consortium. *Cancer Epidemiology, Biomarkers, and Prevention* 18(2):541–550.

Heckley, G. A., J. Jarl, B. O. Asamoah, and U.-G. Gerdtham. 2011. How the risk of liver cancer changes after alcohol cessation: A review and meta-analysis of the current literature. *BMC Cancer* 11:446.

Hendershot, C. S., M. P. Bremmer, M. B. Paladino, G. Kostantinis, T. A. Gilmore, N. R. Sullivan, A. C. Tow, S. S. Dermody, M. A. Prince, R. Jordan, S. A. McKee, P. J. Fletcher, E. D. Claus, and K. R. Klein. 2025. Once-weekly semaglutide in adults with alcohol use disorder: A randomized clinical trial. *JAMA Psychiatry* 82(4):395–405.

Herrnstadt, E., I. W. Parry, and J. Siikamäki. 2015. Do alcohol taxes in Europe and the U.S. rightly correct for externalities? *International Tax and Public Finance* 22:73–101.

Herzog, B., R. Felton, and P. Kanada. 2025. *America's Tobacco: Deep Dive on US Nicotine Market—Who's Best Positioned to Win Over the Next Decade.* New York and London: Goldman Sachs & Co. LLC and Goldman Sachs International.

HHS (Department of Health and Human Services). 1964. *Smoking and health: Report of the Advisory Committee to the Surgeon General of the Public Health Service.* Bethesda, MD: United States Public Health Service Office of the Surgeon General.

HHS. 2014. *The health consequences of smoking—50 years of progress: A report of the surgeon general.* Atlanta, GA: U.S. Department of Health and Human Services, Centers for Disease Control and Prevention.

HHS. 2020a. *Smoking cessation: A report of the surgeon general.* Bethesda, MD: United States Public Health Service Office of the Surgeon General; National Center for Chronic Disease Prevention and Health Promotion, Office on Smoking and Health.

HHS. 2020b. *Treating substance use disorder in older adults.* Treatment improvement protocol (TIP) series no. 26, SAMHSA publication no. Pep20-02-01-011 [preprint]. Rockville, MD: Substance Abuse Mental Health Services Administration, Department of Health and Human Services.

HHS. 2025. *Alcohol and cancer risk: The U.S. surgeon general's advisory.* Bethesda, MD: Office of the Surgeon General, U.S. Department of Health and Human Services.

Hindocha, C., and E. A. McClure. 2021. Unknown population-level harms of cannabis and tobacco co-use: If you don't measure it, you can't manage it. *Addiction* 116(7):1622–1630.

Hurt, R. T., J. O. Ebbert, I. T. Croghan, D. R. Schroeder, R. D. Hurt, and J. T. Hays. 2018. Varenicline for tobacco-dependence treatment in alcohol-dependent smokers: A randomized controlled trial. *Drug and Alcohol Dependence* 184:12–17.

IARC (International Agency for Research on Cancer). 2012. *Personal habits and indoor combustions: IARC monograph on the evaluation of carcinogenic risks to humans.* Lyon, France: International Agency for Research on Cancer.

Inoue-Choi, M., T. S. McNeel, P. Hartge, N. E. Caporaso, B. I. Graubard, and N. D. Freedman. 2019. Non-daily cigarette smokers: Mortality risks in the U.S. *American Journal of Preventive Medicine* 56(1):27–37.

Islami, F., A. Goding Sauer, K. D. Miller, R. L. Siegel, S. A. Fedewa, E. J. Jacobs, M. L. McCullough, A. V. Patel, J. Ma, I. Soerjomataram, W. D. Flanders, O. W. Brawley, S. M. Gapstur, and A. Jemal. 2018. Proportion and number of cancer cases and deaths attributable to potentially modifiable risk factors in the United States. *CA* 68(1):31–54.

Islami, F., E. C. Marlow, B. Thomson, M. L. McCullough, H. Rumgay, S. M. Gapstur, A. V. Patel, I. Soerjomataram, and A. Jemal. 2024. Proportion and number of cancer cases and deaths attributable to potentially modifiable risk factors in the United States, 2019. *CA* 74(5):405–432.

Jernigan, D., J. Noel, J. Landon, N. Thornton, and T. Lobstein. 2017. Alcohol marketing and youth alcohol consumption: A systematic review of longitudinal studies published since 2008. *Addiction* 112 Suppl 1:7–20.

John-Henderson, N. A., E. J. White, and T. L. Crowder. 2023. Resilience and health in American Indians and Alaska Natives: A scoping review of the literature. *Development and Psychopathology* 35(5):2241–2252.

Jordan, A., T. Babuscio, C. Nich, and K. M. Carroll. 2021. A feasibility study providing substance use treatment in the Black church. *Journal of Substance Abuse Treatment* 124:108218.

Kaplan, R. C., S. I. Bangdiwala, J. M. Barnhart, S. F. Castañeda, M. D. Gellman, D. J. Lee, E. J. Pérez-Stable, G. A. Talavera, M. E. Youngblood, and A. L. Giachello. 2014. Smoking among U.S. Hispanic/Latino adults: The Hispanic Community Health Study/Study of Latinos. *American Journal of Preventive Medicine* 46(5):496–506.

Kilian, C., J. M. Lemp, L. Llamosas-Falcón, T. Carr, Y. Ye, W. C. Kerr, N. Mulia, K. Puka, A. M. Lasserre, S. Bright, J. Rehm, and C. Probst. 2023. Reducing alcohol use through alcohol control policies in the general population and population subgroups: A systematic review and meta-analysis. *EClinicalMedicine* 59:101996.

King, A., A. Vena, H. de Wit, J. E. Grant, and D. Cao. 2022. Effect of combination treatment with varenicline and nicotine patch on smoking cessation among smokers who drink heavily: A randomized clinical trial. *JAMA Network Open* 5(3):e220951.

Ling, P. M., and S. A. Glantz. 2002. Why and how the tobacco industry sells cigarettes to young adults: Evidence from industry documents. *American Journal of Public Health* 92(6):908–916.

Ling, P. M., Y. O. Lee, J. Hong, T. B. Neilands, J. W. Jordan, and S. A. Glantz. 2014. Social branding to decrease smoking among young adults in bars. *American Journal of Public Health* 104(4):751–760.

Lortet-Tieulent, J., A. Goding Sauer, R. L. Siegel, K. D. Miller, F. Islami, S. A. Fedewa, E. J. Jacobs, and A. Jemal. 2016. State-level cancer mortality attributable to cigarette smoking in the United States. *JAMA Internal Medicine* 176(12):1792–1798.

Manning, W. G., E. B. Keeler, J. P. Newhouse, E. M. Sloss, and J. Wasserman. 1989. The taxes of sin. Do smokers and drinkers pay their way? *JAMA* 261(11):1604–1609.

McLouth, L. E., B. J. Shelton, V. Bursac, J. L. Burris, J. S. Cheavens, K. Weyman, A. H. Peterman, L. Corum, J. L. Studts, and S. M. Arnold. 2024. "Pathways": A hope-enhancing intervention for patients undergoing treatment for advanced lung cancer. *Psycho-Oncology* 33(3):e6316.

Miech, R. A., L. D. Johnston, M. E. Patrick, P. M. O'Malley, and J. G. Bachman. 2024. *Monitoring the future: National survey results on drug use, 1975–2023: Overview and detailed results for secondary school students*. Institute for Social Research.

Miller, N., T. R. Frieden, S. Y. Liu, T. D. Matte, F. Mostashari, D. R. Deitcher, K. M. Cummings, C. Chang, U. Bauer, and M. T. Bassett. 2005. Effectiveness of a large-scale distribution programme of free nicotine patches: A prospective evaluation. *Lancet* 365(9474):1849–1854.

Moeller, S. J., D. S. Fink, M. Gbedemah, D. S. Hasin, S. Galea, M. J. Zvolensky, and R. D. Goodwin. 2018. Trends in illicit drug use among smokers and nonsmokers in the United States, 2002–2014. *Journal of Clinical Psychiatry* 79(3):17m11718.

Na, P. J., J. Montalvo-Ortiz, I. Petrakis, J. H. Krystal, R. Polimanti, J. Gelernter, and R. H. Pietrzak. 2023. Trajectories of alcohol consumption in U.S. military veterans: Results from a 10-year population-based longitudinal study. *Drug and Alcohol Dependence* 246:109833.

Nargis, N., J. L. Westmaas, E. Orr, M. M. Alqahtani, P. P. Choudhury, F. Islami, and A. Jemal. 2025. Cancer risk and legalisation of access to cannabis in the USA: Overview of the evidence. *Lancet Public Health* 10(2):e160–e164.

NASEM (National Academies of Sciences, Engineering, and Medicine). 2025. *Review of evidence on alcohol and health.* Washington, DC: The National Academies Press.

Nash, S. H., C. Britton, and D. Redwood. 2021. Characteristics of colorectal cancers among Alaska Native people before and after implementing programs to promote screening. *Journal of Cancer Policy* 29:100293.

NCI (National Cancer Institute) and WHO (World Health Organization). 2016. *The economics of tobacco and tobacco control. National Cancer Institute tobacco control monograph 21.* Bethesda, MD: U.S. Department of Health and Human Services, National Institutes of Health, National Cancer Institute; and Geneva, CH: World Health Organization.

Noar, S. M., D. B. Francis, C. Bridges, J. M. Sontag, K. M. Ribisl, and N. T. Brewer. 2016. The impact of strengthening cigarette pack warnings: Systematic review of longitudinal observational studies. *Social Science and Medicine* 164:118–129.

Noel, J. K., T. F. Babor, and K. Robaina. 2017. Industry self-regulation of alcohol marketing: A systematic review of content and exposure research. *Addiction* 112(Suppl 1):28–50.

Palmer, A. M., T. T. Smith, G. J. Nahhas, A. M. Rojewski, B. T. Sanford, M. J. Carpenter, and B. A. Toll. 2021. Interest in quitting e-cigarettes among adult e-cigarette users with and without cigarette smoking history. *JAMA Network Open* 4(4):e214146.

Palmer, A. M., A. M. Rojewski, M. J. Carpenter, E. M. Klemperer, N. L. Baker, B. T. Sanford, and B. A. Toll. 2024. Interest in quitting e-cigarette use by device type and smoking history in US adults. *Tobacco Control* 33(4):537–540.

Palmer, A. M., R. DeMass, A. M. Rojewski, E. M. Bagley, M. J. Carpenter, T. T. Smith, and B. A. Toll. 2025. Augmented doses of nicotine replacement therapy: Feasibility for dual cigarette and e-cigarette cessation. *American Journal of Preventive Medicine*:107664.

Patel, M., B. J. Simard, A. F. Benson, E. M. Donovan, and L. Pitzer. 2023. Measuring the impact of state and local Tobacco 21 policies in the United States: A longitudinal study of youth and young adults ages 15–21. *Nicotine & Tobacco Research* 25(4):631–638.

Pettigrew, S., M. I. Jongenelis, I. S. Pratt, T. Slevin, and T. Chikritzhs. 2017. Drinkers' identification with varying alcohol consumption prototypes. *Drug and Alcohol Review* 36(4):464–467.

Reitsma, M. B., P. J. Kendrick, E. Ababneh, C. Abbafati, M. Abbasi-Kangevari, A. Abdoli, A. Abedi, E. Abhilash, D. B. Abila, and V. Aboyans. 2021. Spatial, temporal, and demographic patterns in prevalence of smoking tobacco use and attributable disease burden in 204 countries and territories, 1990–2019: A systematic analysis from the Global Burden of Disease Study 2019. *The Lancet* 397(10292):2337–2360.

Ribisl, K. M., S. D. Golden, J. Huang, and M. Scollo. 2022. Addressing lower-priced cigarette products through three-pronged comprehensive regulation on excise taxes, minimum price policies and restrictions on price promotions. *Tobacco Control* 31(2):229–234.

Richter, L., B. S. Pugh, P. H. Smith, and S. A. Ball. 2017. The co-occurrence of nicotine and other substance use and addiction among youth and adults in the United States: Implications for research, practice, and policy. *American Journal of Drug and Alcohol Abuse* 43(2):132–145.

Rodriguez, S., N. L. Vanderford, B. Huang, and R. Vanderpool. 2018. A social-ecological review of cancer disparities in Kentucky. *Southern Medical Journal* 111(4):213-219.

Ross, C. S., E. Maple, M. Siegel, W. DeJong, T. S. Naimi, A. A. Padon, D. L. Borzekowski, and D. H. Jernigan. 2015. The relationship between population-level exposure to alcohol advertising on television and brand-specific consumption among underage youth in the US. *Alcohol and Alcoholism* 50(3):358–364.

Rumgay, H., N. Murphy, P. Ferrari, and I. Soerjomataram. 2021a. Alcohol and cancer: Epidemiology and biological mechanisms. *Nutrients* 13(9):3173.

Rumgay, H., K. Shield, H. Charvat, P. Ferrari, B. Sornpaisarn, I. Obot, F. Islami, V. E. P. P. Lemmens, J. Rehm, and I. Soerjomataram. 2021b. Global burden of cancer in 2020 attributable to alcohol consumption: A population-based study. *The Lancet Oncology* 22(8):1071–1080.

Rumgay, H., S. T. Nethan, R. Shah, J. Vignat, O. Ayo-Yusuf, P. Chaturvedi, E. N. S. Guerra, P. C. Gupta, R. Gupta, S. Liu, C. Magnusson, M. Parascandola, Y. C. Paulino, N. Rezaei, K. Siddiqi, S. Warnakulasuriya, B. Lauby-Secretan, and I. Soerjomataram. 2024. Global burden of oral cancer in 2022 attributable to smokeless tobacco and areca nut consumption: A population attributable fraction analysis. *Lancet Oncology* 25(11):1413–1423.

Saad, C., B. H. Cheng, R. Takamizawa, A. Thakur, C. W. Lee, L. Leung, J. L. Veerman, and L. N. Aminde. 2025. Effectiveness of tobacco advertising, promotion and sponsorship bans on smoking prevalence, initiation and cessation: A systematic review and meta-analysis. *Tobacco Control.*

Sanford, B. T., N. C. Brownstein, N. L. Baker, A. M. Palmer, T. T. Smith, A. M. Rojewski, and B. A. Toll. 2024. Shift from smoking cigarettes to vaping nicotine in young adults. *JAMA Internal Medicine* 184(1):106–108.

Sargent, J. D., M. Stoolmiller, H. Dai, J. L. Barrington-Trimis, R. McConnell, J. Audrain-McGovern, and A. M. Leventhal. 2022. First e-cigarette flavor and device type used: Associations with vaping persistence, frequency, and dependence in young adults. *Nicotine and Tobacco Research* 24(3):380–387.

Seidenberg, A. B., K. P. Wiseman, R. H. Eck, K. D. Blake, H. N. Platter, and W. M. P. Klein. 2022. Awareness of alcohol as a carcinogen and support for alcohol control policies. *American Journal of Preventive Medicine* 62(2):174–182.

Seidenberg, A. B., K. P. Wiseman, and W. M. P. Klein. 2023. Do beliefs about alcohol and cancer risk vary by alcoholic beverage type and heart disease risk beliefs? *Cancer Epidemiology, Biomarkers, and Prevention* 32(1):46–53.

Shen, M. J., H. A. Hamann, A. J. Thomas, and J. S. Ostroff. 2016. Association between patient–provider communication and lung cancer stigma. *Supportive Care in Cancer* 24(5):2093–2099.

Spoth, R., M. Greenberg, and R. Turrisi. 2008. Preventive interventions addressing underage drinking: State of the evidence and steps toward public health impact. *Pediatrics* 121(Suppl 4):S311–S336.

Stornetta, A., V. Guidolin, and S. Balbo. 2018. Alcohol-derived acetaldehyde exposure in the oral cavity. *Cancers* 10(1):20.

Thomas, R. E., J. McLellan, and R. Perera. 2015. Effectiveness of school-based smoking prevention curricula: Systematic review and meta-analysis. *BMJ Open* 5(3):e006976.

Toll, B. A., S. Martino, S. S. O'Malley, L. M. Fucito, S. A. McKee, C. W. Kahler, A. M. Rojewski, M. C. Mahoney, R. Wu, P. Celestino, S. Seshadri, J. Koutsky, A. Hyland, and K. M. Cummings. 2015. A randomized trial for hazardous drinking and smoking cessation for callers to a quitline. *Journal of Consulting and Clinical Psychology* 83(3):445–454.

Tommasi, S., H. Blumenfeld, and A. Besaratinia. 2023. Vaping dose, device type, and e-liquid flavor are determinants of DNA damage in electronic cigarette users. *Nicotine and Tobacco Research* 25(6):1145–1154.

Tommasi, S., L. Brocchieri, S. Tornaletti, and A. Besaratinia. 2025. Epigenomic dysregulation in youth vapers: Implications for disease risk assessment. *American Journal of Respiratory Cell and Molecular Biology* 72(2):206–218.

van Amsterdam, J., and W. van den Brink. 2023. The effect of alcohol use on smoking cessation: A systematic review. *Alcohol* 109:13–22.

VanFrank, B., A. Malarcher, M. E. Cornelius, A. Schecter, A. Jamal, and M. Tynan. 2024. Adult smoking cessation—United States, 2022. *MMWR* 73(29):633–641.

Vickers-Smith, R., A. C. Justice, W. C. Becker, C. T. Rentsch, B. Curtis, A. Fernander, E. E. Hartwell, E. T. Ighodaro, R. L. Kember, J. Tate, and H. R. Kranzler. 2023. Racial and ethnic bias in the diagnosis of alcohol use disorder in veterans. *American Journal of Psychiatry* 180(6):426–436.

Warner, K. E., and L. M. Goldenhar. 1985. The cigarette advertising broadcast ban and magazine coverage of smoking and health. *Journal of Public Health Policy* 10(1):32–42.

Warren, G. W., J. R. Marshall, K. M. Cummings, M. A. Zevon, R. Reed, P. Hysert, M. C. Mahoney, A. J. Hyland, C. Nwogu, T. Demmy, E. Dexter, M. Kelly, R. J. O'Connor, T. Houstin, D. Jenkins, P. Germain, A. K. Singh, J. Epstein, K. A. Dobson Amato, and M. E. Reid. 2014a. Automated tobacco assessment and cessation support for cancer patients. *Cancer* 120(4):562–569.

Warren, G. W., S. Sobus, and E. R. Gritz. 2014b. The biological and clinical effects of smoking by patients with cancer and strategies to implement evidence-based tobacco cessation support. *Lancet Oncology* 15(12):e568–e580.

Warren, G. W., K. B. Cartmell, E. Garrett-Mayer, R. G. Salloum, and K. M. Cummings. 2019. Attributable failure of first-line cancer treatment and incremental costs associated with smoking by patients with cancer. *JAMA Network Open* 2(4):e191703.

Warren, G. W., and L. M. Simmons. 2023. Tobacco use and the cancer patient. In *DeVita, Hellman, and Rosenberg's cancer: Principles and practice of oncology*, edited by V. T. DeVita, T. S. Lawrence, and S. A. Rosenberg, 12th ed., 30–42. Philadelphia: Wolters Kluwer.

Waters, E. A., M. T. Kiviniemi, J. L. Hay, and H. Orom. 2022. Dismissing "don't know" responses to perceived risk survey items threatens the validity of theoretical and empirical behavior-change research. *Perspectives on Psychological Science* 17(3):841–851.

Westmaas, J. L., J. Bontemps-Jones, P. S. Hendricks, J. Kim, and L. C. Abroms. 2018. Randomised controlled trial of stand-alone tailored emails for smoking cessation. *Tobacco Control* 27(2):136–146.

White, M. C., D. K. Espey, J. Swan, C. L. Wiggins, C. Eheman, and J. S. Kaur. 2014. Disparities in cancer mortality and incidence among American Indians and Alaska Natives in the United States. *American Journal of Public Health* 104(Suppl 3):S377–S387.

Wiseman, K. P., A. B. Seidenberg, and W. M. P. Klein. 2022. Clinician role in patient awareness regarding carcinogenic nature of alcohol consumption in the U.S.: A nationally representative survey. *Journal of General Internal Medicine* 37(8):2116–2119.

Yammine, L., C. E. Green, T. R. Kosten, C. de Dios, R. Suchting, S. D. Lane, C. D. Verrico, and J. M. Schmitz. 2021. Exenatide adjunct to nicotine patch facilitates smoking cessation and may reduce post-cessation weight gain: A pilot randomized controlled trial. *Nicotine & Tobacco Research* 23(10):1682–1690.

Zhou, H., and V. Vasiliou. 2022. Alcohol use and use disorder and cancer risk: Perspective on causal inference. *Complex Psychiatry* 8(1-2):9–12.

Zhou, H., R. L. Kember, J. D. Deak, H. Xu, S. Toikumo, K. Yuan, P. A. Lind, L. Farajzadeh, L. Wang, A. S. Hatoum, J. Johnson, H. Lee, T. T. Mallard, J. Xu, K. J. A. Johnston, E. C. Johnson, T. T. Nielsen, M. Galimberti, C. Dao, D. F. Levey, C. Overstreet, E. M. Byrne, N. A. Gillespie, S. Gordon, I. B. Hickie, J. B. Whitfield, K. Xu, H. Zhao, L. M. Huckins, L. K. Davis, S. Sanchez-Roige, P. A. F. Madden, A. C. Heath, S. E. Medland, N. G. Martin, T. Ge, J. W. Smoller, D. M. Hougaard, A. D. Børglum, D. Demontis, J. H. Krystal, J. M. Gaziano, H. J. Edenberg, A. Agrawal, H. Zhao, A. C. Justice, M. B. Stein, H. R. Kranzler, J. Gelernter, and Million Veteran Program. 2023a. Multi-ancestry study of the genetics of problematic alcohol use in over 1 million individuals. *Nature Medicine* 29(12):3184–3192.

Zhou, H., B.-Z. Yang, H. Kranzler, and J. Gelernter. 2023b. F101. Mendelian randomization analysis of the effects of alcohol use on cancer risk. Paper presented at the World Congress of Psychiatric Genetics, Montreal, Canada (accessed July 30, 2025).

Zhu, S. H., C. M. Anderson, G. J. Tedeschi, B. Rosbrook, C. E. Johnson, M. Byrd, and E. Gutiérrez-Terrell. 2002. Evidence of real-world effectiveness of a telephone quitline for smokers. *New England Journal of Medicine* 347(14):1087–1093.

Zhu, S. H., E. Aughinbaugh, A. S. Pratt, Y. L. Zhuang, D. Wang, A. Mayoral, C. M. Anderson, and T. Hagaman. 2025. Increasing a quitline's reach to low-income tobacco users through 211 agencies. *Nicotine & Tobacco Research* 27(10):1713–1720.

Zullig, L. L., S. A. Jazowski, N. Chawla, C. D. Williams, D. Winski, C. G. Slatore, A. Clary, K. M. Rasmussen, L. M. Ticknor, and M. J. Kelley. 2024. Summary of Veterans Health Administration cancer data sources. *Journal of Registry Management* 51(1):21–28.

Appendix A

Statement of Task

A National Academies of Sciences, Engineering, and Medicine planning committee will organize and host a 1.5-day public workshop that will explore strategies to reduce tobacco and alcohol use to lower cancer risk and improve health outcomes. The workshop will feature invited presentations and panel discussions on topics that may include

- The effects of tobacco and alcohol use—including synergistic effects—on cancer incidence and outcomes.
- Risk factors for tobacco and alcohol use and their influence on differences in outcomes.
- Clinical practice guidelines, including in the context of cancer treatment, for tobacco cessation and interventions to help patients reduce alcohol use.
- Strategies for data collection and research to address evidence gaps.
- Lessons from tobacco control that could be applied to encourage reduction in alcohol use.
- Impact of recent tobacco policy changes and ways to further advance progress in tobacco control.

The planning committee will develop the agenda for the workshop sessions, select and invite speakers and discussants, and moderate the discussions. A proceedings of the presentations and discussions at the workshop will be prepared by a designated rapporteur in accordance with institutional guidelines.

Appendix B

Workshop Agenda

MARCH 17, 2025

8:30 am **Welcome and Introductory Remarks**
Planning Committee Co-Chairs:
- Roy Herbst, Yale University
- S. Gail Eckhardt, Baylor College of Medicine

8:40 am **Keynote Presentation: Addressing Alcohol and Tobacco and Alcohol Co-Use for Cancer Prevention and Control**
- David Berrigan, National Cancer Institute (Virtual)

A Patient Perspective
- Gwen Darien, Patient Advocate Foundation

9:10 am **Session 1: Overview of Research on the Effects of Tobacco and Alcohol Use on Cancer-Related Health Outcomes**
Co-Moderators:
- Elena Martínez, University of California, San Diego
- S. Gail Eckhardt, Baylor College of Medicine

Overview of Modifiable Risk Factors
- Farhad Islami, American Cancer Society

Epidemiology of Tobacco and Cancer
- Neal Freedman, National Cancer Institute (Virtual)

Epidemiology of Heavy Alcohol Consumption and Cancer
- Jo Freudenheim, University at Buffalo

Global Perspective on the Cancer Burden Attributable to Tobacco and Alcohol Consumption
- Harriet Rumgay, International Agency for Research on Cancer (Virtual)

Research on the Synergistic Effects of Tobacco and Alcohol
- Stephen Hecht, University of Minnesota

Research on the Biological Etiology of Heavy Alcohol Use Disorder
- Hang Zhou, Yale School of Medicine

Indigenous Community Perspective
- Melissa Buffalo, American Indian Cancer Foundation

Panel Discussion
Includes session speakers and
- David Berrigan, National Cancer Institute (Virtual)

10:55 am **Break**

11:10 am **Session 2: Tobacco Control Policy: Lessons Learned and Next Steps**
Co-Moderators:
- Nigar Nargis, American Cancer Society
- Gwen Darien, Patient Advocate Foundation

Overview of Evidence-Based Tobacco Control Policies
- Geoffrey T. Fong, University of Waterloo and Ontario Institute for Cancer Research

Youth Tobacco Prevention and Behavior Change
- Jessica Barrington-Trimis, University of Southern California

Restricting the Sales and Marketing of Tobacco Products to Reduce the Public Health Burden of Tobacco
- Kurt Ribisl, University of North Carolina Gillings School of Global Public Health

Public Health Policy
- Ella Greene-Moton, American Public Health Association (Virtual)

Outcomes of Smoking Cessation Treatment After a Cancer Diagnosis
- Graham Warren, Medical University of South Carolina (Virtual)

Panel Discussion

12:30 pm **Break**

1:30 pm **Session 3: Developing Alcohol Policy: What Is Known, What Can Be Learned from Tobacco Policy, and What's Next?**

Co-Moderators:
- S. Gail Eckhardt, Baylor College of Medicine
- Roy Herbst, Yale University

Price and Taxation of Alcohol: Lessons Learned from Tobacco Policy
- Jeffrey Drope, Johns Hopkins University (Virtual)

Communicating About Alcohol and Cancer Risk: Challenges, Opportunities, and a Way Forward
- Jennifer Hay, Memorial Sloan Kettering Cancer Center

Communication and Awareness
- William Klein, National Cancer Institute (Virtual)

Impact of Marketing on the Youth
- Raimee Eck, Johns Hopkins Bloomberg School of Public Health and Sonrisa Solutions (Virtual)

A Cancer Center's Perspective
- Mark Evers, University of Kentucky Markey Cancer Center

Panel Discussion

3:20 pm **Break**

3:35 pm **Session 4: Evidence-Based Interventions for Tobacco Cessation and to Help Patients Reduce Alcohol Use**
Co-Moderators:
- Roy Jensen, University of Kansas Cancer Center
- Roy Herbst, Yale University

Tailored Email Messages to Help People Quit Smoking: Can It Be Replicated to Help People Quit Heavy Drinking?
- J. Lee Westmaas, American Cancer Society

Quitlines
- Shu-Hong Zhu, University of California, San Diego

Lessons Learned in Tobacco Control in Youth and Young Adults
- Pamela Ling, University of California, San Francisco

Novel Smoking and Vaping Cessation Approaches
- Benjamin Toll, Medical University of South Carolina

Pharmacologic Interventions
- Babalola Faseru, University of Kansas Medical Center

Community Tailored Interventions
- Francisco Cartujano-Barrera, University of Rochester Medical Center
- Ayana Jordan, New York University Grossman School of Medicine (Virtual)

Panel Discussion

5:30 pm **Adjourn**

MARCH 18, 2025

8:30 am **Welcome and Introductory Remarks**
Planning Committee Co-Chair:
- S. Gail Eckhardt, Baylor College of Medicine

8:35 am **Keynote Presentation: Addressing Modifiable Risk Factors Through Public Health Strategies: Lessons from Tobacco**

- Brian King, U.S. Food and Drug Administration

8:55 am **Session 5: Addressing Gaps in Evidence, Practice, and Policy for Tobacco and Alcohol Use**

Co-Moderators:

- Chanita Hughes-Halbert, University of Southern California
- Robert Winn, Massey Comprehensive Cancer Center, Virginia Commonwealth University

Addressing Stigmatization and Perception Bias

- Lisa Carter-Bawa, Cancer Prevention Precision Control Institute, Hackensack Meridian Health Center for Discovery & Innovation

Real-World Experience of Alcohol and Tobacco in a National Health System

- Amy Justice, Yale University; Veterans Affairs Connecticut Healthcare System

Youth-Focused Policy: Differences Between Tobacco and Alcohol

- Adam Leventhal, University of Southern California (Virtual)

Addressing Gaps of Evidence on Moderate Alcohol Consumption and Health

- Ned Calonge, Colorado School of Public Health

Addressing the Gaps in Interventions to Prevent Tobacco Use to Lower Cancer Risk

- Kolawole Okuyemi, Indiana University School of Medicine

Evidence Gaps in Economic Research in Connection with Alcohol Taxation

- Nigar Nargis, American Cancer Society

Panel Discussion

10:25 am **Break**

10:40 am **Session 6: Concluding Discussion and Next Steps**

Co-Moderators:

- S. Gail Eckhardt, Baylor College of Medicine
- Roy Herbst, Yale University

Panelists:

- Session 1: Elena Martínez and S. Gail Eckhardt
- Session 2: Nigar Nargis and Gwen Darien
- Session 3: S. Gail Eckhardt and Roy Herbst
- Session 4: Roy Jensen and Roy Herbst
- Session 5: Chanita Hughes-Halbert and Robert Winn

11:30 am **Adjourn**